PROGRAMME EVALUATION

This book offers a comprehensive, practice-based introduction to conducting effective programme evaluations. It presents the Trident Approach, a three-prong framework focused on outcomes, processes, and stakeholder perspectives that supports robust, real-world evaluations.

Designed for practitioners, policy professionals, managers, and students, this guide walks readers through every stage of the evaluation lifecycle—from identifying needs and formulating questions, to gathering credible data and communicating actionable findings. The book balances methodological guidance with practical tools, case examples, and insights drawn from real evaluation practice. Whether you're seeking to improve service quality, meet accountability demands, fulfil accreditation requirements, or influence policy, this book equips you to conduct evaluations that are credible, useful, and grounded in everyday professional contexts. More than just a technical manual, it fosters a reflective mindset—one committed to learning, integrity, and positive change.

Programme Evaluation: A Practical Guide for Practitioners in Health Care, Social Care and Education is an essential resource for those who wish to use evaluation to generate insight, foster improvement, encourage continuous quality improvement, and support evidence-informed practice.

Roger Ellis is Professor of Applied Psychology at the universities of Ulster and Chester. In 1999, he established the Social and Health Evaluation Unit which has completed more than 100 programme evaluations. He received an Order of the British Empire (OBE) recognising his work in the application of psychology in complex real-life situations including social skill training; quality assurance; and latterly programme evaluation. He has written 15 books dedicated to the communication and utility of psychology.

Elaine Hogard is Professor of Programme Evaluation and Director of Assessment and Programme Evaluation at NOSM University. She has taught and supervised in Canada, the USA, the UK, and has published extensively on programme evaluation theory, method, and practice. Her evaluations span education, health, and social care, emphasising practical applications to complex issues. She is committed to democratising knowledge by ensuring evaluation findings are accessible, meaningful, and useful to practitioners, policymakers, and communities alike.

Programme Evaluation

A Practical Guide for Practitioners in Health Care, Social Care and Education

Roger Ellis and Elaine Hogard

Routledge
Taylor & Francis Group
LONDON AND NEW YORK

Cover image: Connect Images/Getty

First published 2026
by Routledge
4 Park Square, Milton Park, Abingdon, Oxon OX14 4RN

and by Routledge
605 Third Avenue, New York, NY 10158

Routledge is an imprint of the Taylor & Francis Group, an informa business

British Library Cataloguing-in-Publication Data
A catalogue record for this book is available from the British Library

ISBN: 978-1-032-31981-0 (hbk)
ISBN: 978-1-032-31980-3 (pbk)
ISBN: 978-1-003-31225-3 (ebk)

DOI: 10.4324/9781003312253

Typeset in Sabon
by KnowledgeWorks Global Ltd.

Contents

A Trident of Acknowledgements

To all those at the University of Chester who encouraged, supported, and worked with us to develop the Social and Health Evaluation Unit (SHEU).

To those who commissioned our evaluations and had faith in our results.

To those providers and participants who trusted us to do justice to their work and experience.

CHAPTER 1

Introduction

This book is a practical guide intended for use by professional staff in health care, social care, and education. It is based on our 25 years of experience in the Social and Health Evaluation Unit (SHEU) where we undertook more than 100 programme evaluations.

We envisage it being of practical use in three ways. First, it will help in giving insights to those being evaluated. Second, it will help those being evaluated to play a positive part in the evaluation. Third, it will enable professionals to initiate evaluations of their own work or of the work of others.

We need to understand the two words in the title "programme evaluation." In the broad sense, a programme is any organised sequence of activity involving providers and recipients, thus, a half hour workshop or a comprehensive health education initiative could both be described as programmes. Evaluation means posing questions about the programme and gathering evidence to answer them.

We have found it helpful to organise evaluation questions under three broad headings:

1. Outcomes
2. Processes
3. Multiple stakeholder perspectives

We call this the Trident Approach and it is the pervasive theme of this book.

The outcomes are the intended consequences of the programme and are usually expressed in terms of changes of some kind in the recipients' behaviour. They are the reason for the programme and critical in evaluating its success. The process is all in the activities that make up the programme. The multiple stakeholder perspectives are the views of individuals concerned and complement the relatively objective measures of outcomes and process.

Programme evaluations have many benefits but, first and foremost, they provide an objective external view of what the project is achieving, its objectives, and its impact. Second, the evaluation provides evidence of how the programme might

DOI: 10.4324/9781003312253-1

possibly be improved. Third, the report represents a substantial description and evaluation of the programme for those who might wish to emulate it elsewhere. This record on the evaluation could provide evidence for continuation or further funding. Finally, the report might be formulated to produce refereed publications in either or both professional and academic journals.

Thus evaluations can serve multiple purposes, including:

- **Accountability**: Ensuring that resources—funding, time, personnel—are used effectively and ethically.
- **Quality Improvement**: Identifying what works, what doesn't, and how practice can evolve.
- **Influencing Policy and Practice**: Providing evidence that can inform wider strategic or policy directions.
- **Recognition and Celebration**: Capturing successes and recognising the efforts of those involved and applauding those accomplishments.
- **Academic or Professional Publication**: Contributing findings to the broader field through reports or journal articles.

These justifications shape how evaluations are framed, conducted, and shared. Understanding the purpose behind an evaluation is often the first step in initiating it successfully.

THE STARTING POINT: WHAT TRIGGERS AN EVALUATION?

Evaluations typically emerge in response to a need, concern, or opportunity. Understanding these starting points is crucial for practitioners aiming to initiate evaluations that are timely, relevant, and impactful.

Some common triggers include:

- **New Funding**: Many programmes receive evaluation funding as part of grant or contract requirements.
- **Policy Shifts**: Changes in policy often require evidence of effectiveness or alignment with new priorities.
- **Organisational Change**: Structural changes, leadership transitions, or mergers may prompt evaluations to inform new directions.
- **Public or Stakeholder Pressure**: Community groups, service users, or partner organisations may call for evidence of value or performance.
- **Learning Needs**: Internal recognition that more needs to be understood about how a programme is working (or not) often spurs internal or external evaluation efforts.

In practice, these triggers rarely occur in isolation. Often, several converge—for example, a new policy focus combined with increased funding and emerging questions about service delivery.

Tip: When considering initiating an evaluation, begin by asking—what issue, decision, or educational need is prompting this? Clarifying this from the outset helps ensure the evaluation is grounded in real-world relevance.

EARLY DECISIONS: SCOPING THE EVALUATION

Once the need for an evaluation is established, the next step is to scope it—defining its boundaries, priorities, and practical shape.

Key questions include:

- What do we want to find out?
- What aspects of the programme are most critical to explore?
- Who are the key stakeholders?
- What resources (time, budget, personnel) are available?
- What are the timelines and reporting expectations?

An effective evaluation starts with a manageable scope. Trying to evaluate too much at once can lead to superficial findings. A targeted evaluation—focusing, for instance, on a particular process, population, or outcome—often yields deeper insights.

Tip: Use a planning workshop or stakeholder meeting early in the process to identify shared priorities, frame evaluation questions, and build consensus around the evaluation's purpose.

BUILDING A FRAMEWORK: THE TRIDENT APPROACH

The Trident model offers a practical organising framework for evaluation. It consists of three interlinked dimensions:

1. **Outcomes**: What did the programme achieve? This involves measuring changes, impacts, or benefits for participants or systems.
2. **Processes**: How was the programme delivered? This examines the quality, fidelity, efficiency, and reach of implementation.
3. **Stakeholder Perspectives**: What did people involved think of the programme? This includes experiences of participants, staff, and partner organisations.

Using this model ensures the evaluation captures a comprehensive picture—not only whether the programme worked, but how and for whom.

Tip: Even if time or budget limits the evaluation's scope, try to include all three dimensions, even in abbreviated form. Stakeholder perspectives, in particular, often uncovers unanticipated insights.

LAYING THE GROUNDWORK: WHO WILL BE INVOLVED?

Identifying the right participants and roles is essential. Initiating an evaluation is not a solo activity—it requires collaboration and genuine partnerships.

Typical stakeholders may include:

- **Commissioners:** Those who fund or oversee the programme.
- **Managers and Practitioners:** Staff responsible for delivering the programme.
- **Participants or Service Users:** Those who experience the programme first-hand.
- **Partner Organisations:** Collaborating agencies or institutions.
- **Evaluators:** Internal or external individuals conducting the evaluation.

At this stage, clarity around roles and expectations is key. If using an external evaluator, decide whether their role is intended to be more independent (objective, summative) or, *much preferred,* developmental (supportive, formative). Similarly, designate someone to coordinate logistics, data access, and communication.

Tip: Assign a designated contact person to act as a liaison between evaluators and the programme team. This person ensures continuity and facilitates smooth access to data and participants.

BUILDING SUPPORT: GENERATING BUY-IN

Evaluation requires participation, and participation depends on trust. Generating early buy-in is therefore a crucial task.

This can be supported by:

- Clearly explaining the purpose and benefits of the evaluation.
- Being transparent about how findings will be used.
- Ensuring confidentiality and ethical handling of data.
- Involving stakeholders in the design of evaluation questions and methods.
- Showing respect for practitioner and participant time and expertise.
- Demonstrating genuine interest in the project or initiative that is being evaluated.

In many evaluations, initial engagement may be limited, particularly if staff are busy or uncertain about the evaluation's purpose. Personalised outreach, direct communication, relationship building, and reassurance about process and purpose can help overcome this.

Tip: Don't underestimate the value of informal conversations and pre-evaluation meetings. Do not hide how interested you are in the work that is being evaluated. If you don't care—why should they? Real enthusiasm, kindness, and curiosity help build rapport and establish evaluation as a shared endeavour, not an external audit.

MANAGING PRACTICAL CHALLENGES

The early stages of evaluation often involve navigating practical challenges. These may include:

- **Unclear Objectives**: programmes may not have well-defined goals, making it difficult to assess outcomes.
- **Fragmented Data**: Data may exist across multiple systems, in inconsistent formats, or not at all.
- **Conflicting Definitions**: Different stakeholders may define success, participation, or impact differently.
- **Varying Commitment Levels**: Not all stakeholders may be equally invested or available to contribute.

These are not reasons to delay evaluation—they are reasons to design it carefully. Clarifying definitions, creating shared understanding, and identifying achievable goals can transform challenges into opportunities for organisational learning.

Tip: Start with what's feasible. Evaluation doesn't have to be perfect to be useful. Even small, well-focused evaluations can yield valuable applicable insights.

TIMING IS EVERYTHING

The value of evaluation is closely linked to timing. Evaluations conducted too early may lack meaningful data; those undertaken too late may miss critical windows for improvement.

Consider the stage of the programme:

- **Early-Stage** programmes: Best suited to formative evaluations that focus on design, implementation fidelity, and stakeholder feedback.
- **Mid-Stage** programmes: Allow for interim evaluations that assess early outcomes and adjust delivery.
- **Mature** programmes: Suitable for summative evaluations that focus on long-term impact and strategic planning.

Evaluations should also be timed with key decision points—such as renewal, scaling, or redesign—so that findings can directly inform choices.

Tip: If you're unsure whether it's "too early" to evaluate, consider starting with a process evaluation. Understanding how things are working is a crucial first step to understanding what outcomes may result.

MAKING RECOMMENDATIONS USEFUL

The outcome of a good evaluation is not just a report—it's actionable insight. From the beginning, consider how findings will be used and by whom.

Key practices include:

- **Linking Findings to Decisions**: Tailor recommendations to current planning, funding, or strategic processes.
- **Clarifying Next Steps**: Include not just what should be done, but how and by whom.
- **Celebrating Progress**: Recognise what is working well, and also, areas for change.
- **Tailoring Communication**: Use summaries, infographics, or presentations as appropriate for your audience.

Tip: Think beyond reports. A workshop with stakeholders to discuss findings can be more effective than pages of written documentation alone.

CONCLUSION: A STARTING PLACE FOR LEARNING

Evaluations begin not with data but with a question. They start when individuals or organisations decide that understanding is better than assumption; that evidence is more powerful than speculation. This chapter has aimed to demystify the early stages of that process.

Whether prompted by policy, funding, concern, or curiosity, evaluations are part of a broader learning culture. Initiating them thoughtfully—by clarifying purpose, involving the right people, and designing within your resources—lays the groundwork for useful and credible findings.

In summary, the essential steps in initiating a programme evaluation are:

1. **Identify the need or trigger** for evaluation.
2. **Clarify the purpose**—what do you want to know and why?
3. **Engage key stakeholders** early in the process.
4. **Define your evaluation questions** using a model like the Trident.
5. **Map your available data** and resources.
6. **Assign roles** for coordination and communication.
7. **Secure buy**-in through transparency and shared goals.
8. **Be practical and flexible**—start small if needed but do start.
9. **Plan for use**—ensure findings will inform real decisions.
10. **Celebrate the process**—evaluation is a step forward in itself and enthusiasm is infectious.

With a clear beginning, the path of evaluation becomes not only manageable but truly interesting and ultimately meaningful.

Programme evaluations tend to follow a similar sequence from conception to the production of the report and implementation of its recommendations. This constitutes a typical life history for a programme evaluation and the next chapter goes through these stages. Remaining chapters focus primarily on our Trident method looking in detail at evaluation questions and ways to gather data to address them and final chapters of guidance on report writing; recommendations on the implementation and subsequent publications in professional and academic journals. Finally, we consider programme evaluation as a key element in Continuous Quality Improvement.

Integrating with the chapters are our summaries of reports from the SHEU demonstrating the Trident in action. Our intention for this book, from the start, was to include both advice to implement the Trident Approach and examples of the Trident in Action in the form of summaries of SHEU reports. In the end, we have decided to integrate the reports with the expository chapters. We hope this is illuminating but does not obscure the particular topics of chapters. We believe the integrated reports are relevant not only to the individual chapters but to the Trident Approach generally and thus all chapters.

CHAPTER 2

The life history of a programme evaluation

A practical guide from a case study of a complex multi-site community programme

INTRODUCTION

Programme evaluation is best understood not as a fixed, one-time activity, but as a dynamic process with a distinct life history. From inception to completion, evaluations tend to follow a sequence of interrelated stages that reflect the evolving needs of funders, service providers, participants, communities, and policy environments. This chapter outlines those stages, offering an integrated view of the evaluation process grounded in both practical experience and methodological guidance.

Evaluations are often initiated as conditions of funding or as part of internal quality assurance and continuous improvement. Whether externally mandated or internally driven, the purpose of evaluation remains consistent: to pose meaningful questions about a programme and gather evidence to answer them. This demands a logical framework—such as the Trident Approach used in this book—that organises questions around outcomes, processes, and stakeholder perspectives.

Each stage of the evaluation entails distinct tasks with clear objectives, deliverables, and responsibilities. Interim and final reports serve not only as records of findings but as vehicles for actionable recommendations. These reports may also form the basis for professional and academic dissemination.

By presenting a detailed case study of a complex multi-site community initiative, this chapter illustrates how the life history of an evaluation unfolds in practice. It provides a practical roadmap for navigating the complexity of evaluating multi-agency community-driven programmes but also a guide for more straightforward initiatives and sets the stage for the expanded direction offered in subsequent chapters.

DOI: 10.4324/9781003312253-2

STARTING POINTS

Every evaluation begins in a particular social and political context. In the example drawn from this programme, the initiative was launched in response to a national policy agenda focused on reducing child poverty, improving early childhood development, and strengthening family support in areas of concentrated deprivation. The decision to initiate an evaluation was itself shaped by these policy imperatives, as well as the need for local accountability and continuous quality improvement.

The case study area faced serious structural challenges, including high unemployment, poor health outcomes, and a large number of lone-parent households. These conditions provided both the rationale for intervention and a baseline against which future progress could be assessed. Evaluation thus began not with data collection, but with understanding the programme's origins, values, and intended contributions.

Practical Tip: Always begin an evaluation by articulating the socio-political origins of the programme. Examine the funding mechanisms, community needs assessments, and strategic policy drivers that justified the intervention. This foundational step ensures the evaluation remains grounded in real-world conditions.

PRELIMINARY QUESTIONS

Following the recognition of the need for evaluation, the next phase involves the formulation of preliminary questions. These questions are not yet tightly defined indicators, but rather, thematic lines of inquiry that help determine the scope and focus of the evaluation.

In this initiative, key questions included: are services reaching the intended families? How do community members perceive their involvement in decision-making? What kinds of changes are visible in family wellbeing? These preliminary questions emerged from early conversations with programme staff, parents, and partner agencies. They were also influenced by national guidance from the central evaluation support body, which emphasised implementation fidelity, stakeholder engagement, and long-term impact.

Practical Tip: Begin by gathering informal feedback and mapping key concerns across different stakeholder groups. Use this to formulate roughly four to six broad themes that your evaluation should address. Don't rush into measurement before you've defined what matters most locally.

PARTNERSHIP AND STEERING GROUP

A vital component of the evaluation's life history is the establishment of a robust governance and partnership structure. In the case study, this was achieved through a multi-agency steering group composed of programme staff, parents, representatives from local schools, health services, and evaluation professionals.

The steering group played multiple roles: approving data collection plans, facilitating access to participants, interpreting findings, and ensuring that the evaluation remained responsive to community priorities. Importantly, this group met regularly throughout the evaluation process and served as both a sounding board and accountability mechanism.

Notably, the inclusion of parents in governance roles was central to the programme's ethos. Parents participated not only in focus groups but also on management boards and subcommittees, bringing real-time insight into how the programme affected family life.

Practical Tip: Form a steering group early and ensure that it includes end-users (e.g., parents, service participants) alongside professionals. Clarify the group's role in decision-making and data interpretation. *Empower the group to challenge and reshape evaluation plans if and when needed.*

EVALUATION QUESTIONS AND DATA STREAMS

As the evaluation matured, the preliminary questions were refined into more specific evaluation questions. These were organised using the Trident framework: outcomes, processes, and stakeholder perspectives. Each prong of the Trident required distinct data sources and analytical strategies.

For outcomes, the evaluation relied on longitudinal data from parental satisfaction surveys, health records, and programme usage statistics. For process, documentation of how services were delivered—especially the rollout of the new roles and services —provided critical evidence of adaptation and innovation. Stakeholder perspectives were captured through in-depth interviews with service users, staff, and referral agencies.

For example, data showed that average family registration with the programme nearly doubled over a period while the proportion of "hard-to-reach" families engaging with services had also increased. Parents described the programme as transformative, citing access to mental health support, parenting classes, and community playgroups as central to their improved wellbeing.

Practical Tip: Design your evaluation questions in alignment with available and collectable data. Be clear about which questions require quantitative versus qualitative responses. *Use the Trident model to ensure balance across different domains of inquiry.*

OVERALL DESIGN AND STRUCTURE: THE EVALUATION TRIDENT

The Trident model offers a comprehensive yet flexible structure for organising evaluation. In the case study, this model allowed the team to avoid overemphasising outcomes at the expense of understanding how change occurred or how it was experienced.

For instance, an outcome-only approach might have celebrated improved survey scores in parental satisfaction, but the process component of the evaluation revealed that satisfaction plateaued in later years as parental expectations rose. This was a vital insight: success had raised the community's standards and future services would need to evolve accordingly.

The stakeholder component of the Trident added further depth. Parents did not just use services; they co-designed them. Their critiques and suggestions shaped everything from service delivery hours to the content of parenting courses.

Practical Tip: Treat the Trident model not as three separate tasks but as an integrated evaluation architecture. Build feedback loops between the three prongs—how outcomes prompt new processes and how stakeholder voices reshape goals all in order to tease out possible relationships and any cause and effects in the programme.

PROJECT MANAGEMENT AND RESPONSIBILITIES

Evaluation is not only about methods and findings—it is also a project that must be managed effectively. In the case example, the evaluation team implemented a phased work plan with clear timelines, deliverables, and responsibilities. This included timelines for ethics approval, data collection, interim reports, and final synthesis.

Challenges included delayed access to health records, the need to re-schedule fieldwork due to staff turnover, and adjustments to data tools in response to community feedback. These were handled by maintaining close communication with the steering group and remaining flexible in approach.

Practical Tip: Assign a project manager or coordinator for the evaluation. Maintain a risk log and contingency plans. Establish clear reporting routines—monthly updates to programme leadership and quarterly formal reports to the steering group to stay on track.

OUTCOMES

Outcomes were at the centre of the evaluation. The evaluation documented tangible improvements in service uptake, family functioning, and early childhood development. These included:

- A substantial rise in families registered with the programme which doubled over the course of the initiative.
- Statistically significant improvements in parental satisfaction scores, especially in areas such as perceived access to support and quality of early education provision.
- Evidence of parental progression to employment or volunteering roles within the programme itself.

The evaluation also tracked the performance of certain interventions. For instance, specific services were credited by parents with preventing family crises and providing crucial emotional support.

Practical Tip: Don't limit outcome measurement to hard indicators. Include qualitative indicators of change—stories, testimonials, and perceived differences in wellbeing. These add genuine depth and life to the numbers.

PROCESS

Process evaluation revealed how the programme developed a culture distinct from statutory services. Staff recruitment prioritised commitment to the programme's ethos—flexibility, respect, and non-hierarchical teamwork. The service delivery model emphasised accessibility, with flexible hours, mobile workers, and non-clinical settings.

Key insights included the use of community assets like refurbished buildings and local partnerships (e.g., colleges offering parenting courses) to embed services within the neighbourhood. This contrasted with centralised statutory models which were often perceived as impersonal and rigid.

Practical Tip: Document both formal and informal processes. Track how decisions are made, how services adapt over time, and how clients are referred and engaged. Use observational data where possible to capture delivery in action.

MULTIPLE STAKEHOLDER PERSPECTIVES

Stakeholder involvement was a hallmark of the programme. In addition to structured surveys and interviews, the evaluation used participatory methods, including parent-led focus groups and workshops where findings were co-analysed.

Diverse perspectives emerged. Staff spoke of the joy and pressure of working in a dynamic, experimental environment. Parents highlighted their dual role as service users and co-producers. External partners offered insights into how the programme modelled a new form of inter-agency collaboration.

Practical Tip: Involve stakeholders in interpreting the data. Don't just extract opinions; co-construct meaning. Where possible, use visual tools (e.g., charts, storyboards) to facilitate engagement across literacy levels.

REPORTING

The evaluation produced multiple reports tailored to different audiences. Strategic summary reports were created for funders and policymakers. Detailed thematic reports (e.g., on buildings, service usage, parental involvement) were shared with programme staff. A final integrated report synthesised findings and was used for dissemination nationally.

Efforts were made to present data in accessible formats—using infographics, quotes, and straightforward charts. Reporting was not seen as the end but as part of an ongoing dialogue about improvement.

Practical Tip: Don't write just one final report. Think in terms of multiple products: executive summaries, policy briefs, community newsletters, and academic papers. Build communication into your timeline from the outset.

IMPACT ON POLICY AND PRACTICE

The evaluation's influence was visible in multiple domains. Locally, it led to increased funding for successful interventions, a redesign of staff training, and greater parental involvement in service design. At the regional level, findings were presented at strategic meetings to inform rollout of similar programmes elsewhere.

The greatest legacy was cultural: a shift in how services were understood—not as something delivered to families but cooperatively with them.

Practical Tip: Follow-up after the final report. Track how findings are being used. Offer additional sessions or workshops to help translate evaluation into action. *Real influence and impact often comes post-report.*

PUBLICATION AND RESEARCH

Finally, the evaluation contributed to the wider evidence base. Findings were shared through academic presentations, policy seminars, and practitioner forums. Ethical considerations around anonymity, informed consent, and community ownership of data were strictly observed.

Importantly, the process of publication reinforced the credibility of the programme and the legitimacy of community voices.

Practical Tip: Build dissemination into your evaluation budget and timeline. Include community authors or co-presenters where appropriate. Ensure findings return to those who contributed their time and experience.

CONCLUSION

The life history of a programme evaluation is more than a methodological exercise—it is a story of relationships, learning, and layered change. As the case study of this initiative shows, evaluations that are grounded, participatory, and theoretically robust can shape both the programmes they assess and the systems in which they support. By following the 12 stages outlined here, evaluators can approach their work not as detached analysts but as co-inquirers in a collective effort to improve lives.

CHAPTER 3

The Trident

Implementing the evaluation Trident using a case study in the development of a new healthcare support role

In this chapter, we look in more depth at our organising model for programme evaluation which we call the Trident as it focuses evaluation questions and data gathering to answer them under the three main headings:

1. Outcomes
2. Processes
3. Multiple stakeholder perspectives

We started our first programme evaluation back in 1999 asking stakeholders for evaluation questions they felt we should attempt to answer within the evaluation. It quickly became clear that the questions were mainly of two types: addressing if the programme worked? And how did the programme work?

Typical questions in the first category were:

- Did the programme work?
- Did the programme meet its objectives?
- Did the programme achieve what it promised?
- What happened at the end of the programme?

Typical questions in the second category were:

- How did the programme work?
- What did the professionals do? What were the participants doing in the programme?
- What details were provided in and by the programme?
- What, when, and where was the programme happening?

DOI: 10.4324/9781003312253-3

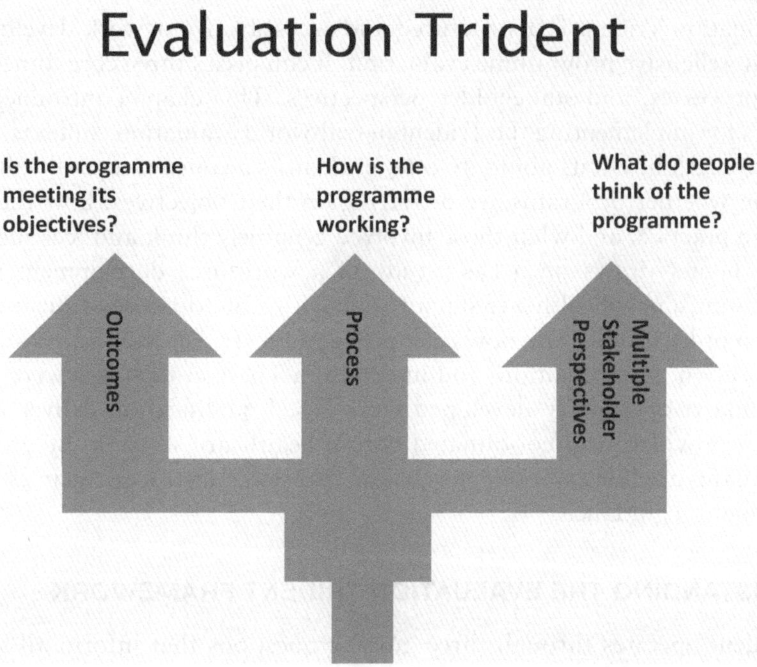

FIGURE 3.1 Evaluation Trident

We called these groupings of questions: outcomes and processes. It is important not to confuse process variables with outcomes. While aspects of delivery are, of course objectives, they are not outcomes of the programme, but features of the programme.

The evidence for achieving outcomes must measure up to scientific standards of validity and reliability and should, were possible, be quantitative in nature. The description of the process and its variables should also measure up to scientific standards of replicability.

In considering outcomes and processes, it is important that the answer to questions should be objective and external. However, it is clear that participant perceptions are not the same as their behaviour and we felt it was important to capture the phenomenology of a programme, in other words, the perceptions of participants and providers. This led to a third prong for the Trident which we have called Multiple Stakeholder Perspectives. While the evidence regarding stakeholders' perceptions can be as objective and quantitative, as that for outcomes and processes, it is more likely to be qualitative in nature.

Thus the use of the Trident requires mixed method for its balance of objectivity and subjective validity.

The formulation of evaluation questions and the gathering of evidence to address them for each of the prongs of the Trident (figure 3.1) are covered in subsequent chapters.

CASE STUDY IN THE DEVELOPMENT OF A NEW HEALTHCARE SUPPORT ROLE

The Evaluation Trident is a structured and accessible framework developed to support comprehensive programme evaluation. It comprises three core dimensions: outcomes, processes, and stakeholder perspectives. This chapter introduces practical strategies for implementing the Trident in real-world evaluation contexts. The framework's strength lies in its ability to offer evaluators a consistent yet flexible means of exploring whether programs are delivering on their objectives, how they are functioning in practice, and what those involved genuinely think and feel about them.

This chapter draws on a case study of a workforce development programme implementing a new healthcare support role with a multi-agency educational collaboration in order to illustrate how each prong of the Trident can be explored through data collection, interpretation, and integration. These evaluations were undertaken in the context of a newly developed work-based qualification delivered jointly by education providers and coordinated within healthcare services. By grounding the Trident in this applied example, the chapter translates abstract principles into actionable evaluation guidance.

UNDERSTANDING THE EVALUATION TRIDENT FRAMEWORK

The Trident operates through three guiding questions that inform all stages of an evaluation, from planning to reporting. The first question addresses whether the programme is achieving its intended outcomes. The second explores how the programme is being delivered and what processes underpin or hinder its operation. The third focuses on the views and experiences of all stakeholders involved in the programme—participants, providers, partners, and funders.

These lines of inquiry are mutually reinforcing. Understanding outcomes without understanding the processes behind them risks shallow analysis, while ignoring stakeholder perspectives can result in missed learning and disengaged participants. By intentionally balancing all three, the Trident supports well-rounded and developmentally useful evaluations.

INVESTIGATING OUTCOMES: ASSESSING PROGRAMME SUCCESS

One of the central pillars of the Trident involves identifying and assessing the degree to which a programme is achieving its intended results. In the context of the health education programme, evaluators began by defining core objectives around student recruitment, course completion, and the enhancement of professional career pathways for support staff. Evaluators gathered data from institutional records, surveys, and interviews to create a profile of students enrolling in a new degree aimed at developing healthcare practitioners.

Outcome data revealed a number of encouraging trends. The programme had succeeded in attracting a diverse cohort, with a significant proportion of students coming from non-traditional educational backgrounds. Most of the learners had prior work experience in health settings, although their educational qualifications varied widely. The course clearly addressed a gap in the career progression pathway for many participants, offering formal recognition for skills previously acquired on the job. Students expressed strong motivation to use the programme as a stepping stone—some aimed for further academic study, while others looked forward to promotion within their service areas.

However, outcome evaluation also revealed challenges. While enrolment numbers were strong, the evaluation noted regional imbalances in recruitment, with some areas under-represented. This pointed to the need for improved marketing and coordination with regional employers.

In this instance, outcomes were not measured solely in terms of completion rates or qualifications awarded. Equally important were students' aspirations, confidence levels, and career intentions. Interviews revealed that many participants had long been overlooked for advancement due to a lack of formal credentials. The course allowed them to re-enter education in a manageable way, supported by workplace placements and employer backing. Evaluators found that the programme met a significant need for validation and recognition among existing staff, and that this outcome—although not explicitly planned—was highly valuable.

To assess such complex outcomes, evaluators must combine quantitative metrics with qualitative insights. Administrative data can track enrolment and completion, but it is only through interviews and narrative responses that the depth of personal transformation becomes visible. For future evaluators, the key takeaway is to *approach outcomes as multi-dimensional, extending beyond the programme's formal objectives to encompass unanticipated but meaningful results.*

EVALUATING PROCESSES: WHAT IS ACTUALLY HAPPENING IN DELIVERY?

The process prong of the Trident directs evaluators to examine how a programme is functioning on the ground. In this case, the delivery of the degree was coordinated across three higher education institutions working in collaboration with a public health authority. This multi-agency configuration required not only logistical coordination but also a shared understanding of goals, responsibilities, and decision-making protocols.

To explore how this partnership operated in practice, evaluators used a collaborative measurement framework. This framework assessed key attributes of effective collaboration, including shared purpose, trust, commitment, governance structures, and monitoring mechanisms. Data collection included questionnaires completed by both operational staff and strategic leaders, supplemented by focus groups and individual interviews.

Findings showed that while operational-level collaboration was generally strong—characterised by mutual respect, regular communication, and shared effort—strategic-level partnerships faced more significant tensions. Disagreements about student number allocations, leadership roles, and decision-making authority created some discord between institutions. A few partners described the collaboration as externally imposed and questioned whether a genuine partnership could flourish under conditions of competition and unclear accountability.

These process findings were crucial in explaining the challenges encountered during programme implementation. For instance, delays in course validation, inconsistent student recruitment timelines, and fragmented communication between institutions were all partially attributable to process weaknesses. Evaluators recommended clearer contractual arrangements, more transparent allocation of leadership, and the establishment of a neutral convenor to oversee joint governance. These were findings that would not have emerged through outcome data alone.

A practical lesson for evaluators is the value of disaggregating the "how" at multiple levels. It is not enough to ask whether the programme was delivered—it is essential to ask how decisions were made, who held responsibility for what, and whether the systems in place were conducive to timely and effective implementation.

In the context of the case study, process evaluation also highlighted the strengths of collaborative curriculum design. Despite organisational tensions, academic staff across institutions managed to validate a joint qualification that was consistent across sites and responsive to sector needs. This success pointed to the potential of future joint design processes when supported by clear parameters and mutual respect.

Thus, process evaluation revealed both obstacles and enablers. It offered a textured picture of what worked and what required refinement. For complex programs, particularly those involving multiple institutions or agencies, attention to process is not optional—it is fundamental to understanding how and why outcomes are achieved.

CAPTURING STAKEHOLDER PERSPECTIVES: LISTENING TO THE PEOPLE INVOLVED

Stakeholder perspectives are the third essential dimension of the Trident. In this case study and in all others, considerable effort was made to collect the views of those at the heart of the programme—learners, academic staff, managers, and organisational leaders. Their insights enriched the evaluation and unearthed key issues that might otherwise have been overlooked.

For students, entering higher education was often a daunting but exciting step. Interviews revealed that many had not studied formally in years and expressed anxiety about assessments, academic expectations, and balancing work, study, and home life. Nonetheless, students valued the opportunity to progress without needing to leave their current roles or workplaces. The programme's flexible structure—allowing in-service learning and departmental placements—was repeatedly cited as a strength. One student described the relief of studying in a familiar work environment noting that it reduced the stress of transition and enhanced relevance.

These perspectives were not merely anecdotal. They provided insight into student retention, engagement, and potential barriers to success. For example, several students reported that the speed of the recruitment and enrolment process left them underprepared. Others commented on the lack of accessible course information prior to starting. These findings directly informed recommendations around streamlining recruitment timelines, improving communication, and tailoring pre-course induction for adult learners.

Staff perspectives also added value. Academic leads discussed the challenges of working with differing institutional policies, assessment systems, and timetables. While committed to the joint programme, some described difficulties coordinating curriculum development and ensuring parity across sites. Their reflections pointed to the need for institutional flexibility and the development of shared quality assurance processes.

From a managerial standpoint, perspectives varied. Operational managers tended to focus on problem-solving and delivery, often expressing pride in the cross-institutional teamwork. Strategic leaders, by contrast, were more circumspect. Some questioned whether the partnership model could be sustained long-term, given the competitive funding environment. This difference in outlook—optimism at the front line, uncertainty at the top—highlighted an important dynamic. Evaluators were able to use this insight to recommend alignment mechanisms such as joint strategy sessions and cross-level planning reviews.

A key learning point is that *stakeholder perspectives should be gathered early, often, and across roles*. Surveys alone are insufficient; in-depth interviews, group discussions, and reflective exercises add nuance and depth. Moreover, capturing dissenting views is just as important as confirming success stories. Evaluations that silence critical voices risk presenting a distorted picture, undermining credibility and utility.

INTEGRATING THE TRIDENT: BUILDING A COHERENT PICTURE

Although the Trident is organised around three distinct dimensions, its strength lies in their integration. In practice, outcomes, processes, and perspectives overlap and influence each other. A robust evaluation will not only explore each dimension but will also map how they interact.

In this case, integration occurred in several ways. For instance, outcome data showing high student motivation was contextualised by interview findings that revealed career stagnation and a desire for progression. Similarly, the achievement of curriculum validation was understood more deeply through process evaluation, which illuminated the behind-the-scenes work of operational staff navigating competing institutional demands.

By connecting the dots, evaluators constructed a coherent narrative: a programme that met a clear workforce need, delivered strong short-term results, but was vulnerable to structural tensions in its governance. This narrative enabled recommendations that were both specific and systemic—calling for changes in recruitment procedures, curriculum induction, and inter-agency governance.

Evaluators using the Trident should structure their reporting to reflect this integration. Rather than separating each dimension into siloed sections, interweaving findings enables richer insight. For example, a report might begin with a headline outcome—such as high enrolment rates—then explore the process conditions that supported it and the perspectives that give it meaning. This approach enhances readability and fosters understanding.

REFLECTIONS AND RECOMMENDATIONS FOR PRACTICE

Implementing the Evaluation Trident requires attentiveness, balance, and methodological pluralism. The model's value lies in its adaptability across contexts and its insistence on seeing programs as more than the sum of their outputs.

Evaluators embarking on new projects should begin by designing data collection strategies aligned with all three Trident dimensions. Early engagement with programme planners and delivery staff can help shape appropriate tools—be they interviews, surveys, observational methods, or document reviews. Crucially, the evaluation should remain open to emergent findings, adjusting focus if stakeholder concerns or unforeseen outcomes arise.

Furthermore, evaluators should guard against overemphasis on one prong at the expense of others. A focus solely on outcomes, for example, may miss critical delivery challenges. Likewise, a rich exploration of perspectives means little if unaccompanied by analysis of what was actually achieved. *The Trident helps ensure such balance is maintained.*

Finally, evaluators must communicate findings in accessible, grounded language. In the case studies described, clear reporting led to concrete changes in programme delivery. Students received better information. Managers adjusted recruitment timelines. Institutions reviewed their governance structures. These are signs of evaluation that matters, not just for funders or academic audiences, but for the people whose lives and work are shaped by the programs being assessed.

CONCLUSION

The Evaluation Trident is a powerful model for structuring and delivering meaningful programme evaluations. Its three-pronged approach—focusing on outcomes, processes, and stakeholder perspectives—ensures evaluations are comprehensive, inclusive, and responsive to real-world complexity. When applied with care and insight, as shown in the case study featured in this chapter, it supports learning, improvement, and accountability across diverse settings.

Whether working in health, education, community development, or beyond, evaluators can rely on the Trident as a practical and adaptable framework. It not only guides inquiry but promotes reflexivity and balance—helping ensure that evaluations do justice to the ambitions, challenges, and lived experiences of those participating.

CHAPTER 4

Establishing the starting point of a programme evaluation

As mentioned in Chapter 2, programme evaluations may have various starting points. A programme evaluation may be externally driven or required by the programme's organisation or initiated by the programme itself. Understanding how and why a programme evaluation begins is a critical first step in designing a meaningful and responsive evaluation. As outlined in earlier chapters, evaluations may be initiated for a range of reasons—externally imposed, internally motivated, or as a hybrid of both. This chapter explores these varied starting points and uses a case study to demonstrate how an evaluation was shaped by its origins.

WHY EVALUATIONS ARE INITIATED

Programme evaluations do not occur in a vacuum. Their design, focus, and implementation are shaped by the motivations and expectations of their initiators. These motivations can generally be grouped into two broad categories: externally driven and internally initiated evaluations.

EXTERNALLY DRIVEN EVALUATIONS

In many instances, programme evaluations are mandated by external bodies—such as funding agencies, regulatory authorities, or policymakers—as a condition of support. Competitive funding processes often require recipients to demonstrate that public or private monies are being used effectively and for their intended purposes. In such cases, the evaluation becomes a mechanism of accountability, providing assurance to funders that investments are justified and results are measurable.

An important feature of externally required evaluations is that they are often embedded into the terms of the funding agreement. For example, one of the earliest evaluations undertaken by our team involved a programme in which 10% of the total project budget was earmarked specifically for evaluation activities. This allocation

DOI: 10.4324/9781003312253-4

was non-negotiable and reflected a wider trend in public funding frameworks that require demonstrable outcomes and rigorous scrutiny of resource use.

External evaluations also serve additional strategic purposes. A well-executed evaluation can enhance the visibility of a programme, offering a form of legitimacy and validation. The final report—often disseminated widely—can contribute to public discourse, inform policy, and support further bids for funding.

INTERNALLY INITIATED EVALUATIONS

Not all evaluations are externally mandated. Many are initiated by the programme organisation itself as part of a proactive approach to learning, development, and continuous quality assurance. These evaluations tend to be more formative in nature, often designed to explore processes, understand implementation barriers, or compare the current intervention with past models or sector benchmarks.

Organisations may choose to initiate such evaluations as part of a culture of continuous improvement. Rather than waiting for external requirements, they embed evaluation into their practice as a developmental tool. This kind of evaluation may focus on identifying what is working well, uncovering areas for improvement, and building evidence to support internal decision-making.

Internally driven evaluations tend to be more flexible and responsive to context. They can adapt to emerging issues, support organisational learning, and build evaluation capacity within teams. While they may lack the formal pressure of externally mandated evaluations, they can be equally robust and insightful when properly resourced and supported.

A CASE STUDY FRAMING: WHERE THE EVALUATION BEGAN

In this case study, the evaluation was initiated under conditions that illustrate a common blend of external and internal motivations. The programme under review had secured competitive funding from a national initiative aimed at promoting innovation in public services. As part of the grant agreement, the funder stipulated that a percentage of the budget be allocated to independent evaluation. This external requirement provided the formal trigger for evaluation activity.

However, the organisation hosting the programme had its own internal motivations for seeking an evaluation. Having previously implemented similar initiatives, the organisation was interested in comparing outcomes, identifying improvements in delivery mechanisms, and assessing cost-effectiveness relative to earlier models. The organisation also wanted to use the findings as part of a longer-term strategic planning process and to strengthen its reputation as a learning-focused and results-oriented institution.

This dual-purpose evaluation—externally required but internally valued—shaped the evaluation design from the outset. It required careful negotiation of priorities between funders, programme staff, and evaluators. An evaluation steering group was formed, bringing together key stakeholders to guide the process, set expectations, and ensure that both accountability and learning objectives were met.

SETTING THE EVALUATION IN MOTION

Once the rationale for evaluation was established, the next step was to design a process that reflected both funder requirements and internal organisational goals. The role of the evaluation team was to translate these expectations into a clear plan: one that included interim reporting milestones, regular communication with the steering group, and a final report capable of addressing both accountability and improvement.

The early establishment of a steering group proved essential. Composed of representatives from the funder, programme staff, and independent evaluators, this group provided strategic oversight, clarified expectations, and helped resolve any tensions between different perspectives. Interim reports were reviewed by the group, allowing for timely feedback, adjustments in evaluation focus, and the co-construction of findings. The final report, when delivered, had both credibility and utility across the range of stakeholders.

LESSONS FOR PRACTICE

For practitioners looking to undertake or commission a programme evaluation, understanding the starting point is essential. The origin of the evaluation—whether external or internal—will shape:

- Evaluation Questions: What is being asked, and why?
- Design and Methods: What approaches are feasible and appropriate?
- Timing and Resources: What constraints and expectations exist?
- Stakeholder Engagement: Who needs to be involved, and at what stages?

Whether an evaluation begins as a contractual obligation or as a voluntary act of organisational learning, clarity about its rationale helps set realistic goals and fosters a more constructive evaluation process. Ideally, both internal and external stakeholders find value in the process, leading to improved practice, strengthened accountability, and informed decision-making.

HOW TO BEGIN A PROGRAMME EVALUATION: PRACTICAL INSIGHTS USING A CASE STUDY APPROACH WITH A HOSPITAL BASED APPLIED HEALTH PRACTICE AND RESEARCH CENTRE (AHPRC)

Introduction: Understanding evaluation starting points

Programme evaluations do not emerge in a void; they begin in response to real-world questions, needs, and pressures. As outlined in the "Starting Points" framework, evaluations are commonly initiated due to external or internal imperatives, ranging from compliance with funding conditions to internal aspirations for quality improvement. Each origin point shapes the scope and intent of the evaluation. This section explores how such starting points are operationalized through a practical case study—an anonymized hospital-based applied health practice and research centre—to illustrate how these motivations directly influence the design, methods, and focus of an evaluation.

External-Internal Continuum: A framework for origins

The proposal document establishes an External–Internal Continuum to map the motivations behind initiating evaluations. At the external end lie mandatory evaluations, often tied to funding or accountability requirements. Internally driven evaluations emerge from managerial or professional interests in learning and improving. This spectrum helps evaluators clarify the evaluative stance and purpose.

In the case of the hospital AHPRC evaluation, the origin sits closer to the internal end of the continuum. The initiative emerged from within the healthcare setting, motivated by a desire to improve practice, foster a culture of inquiry, and build collaborative links with a higher education partner. This positioning influenced the evaluation's focus: assessing the effectiveness of processes, staff development outcomes, and stakeholder experiences, rather than merely fulfilling external accountability criteria.

Programme evaluation as a condition of funding

One common starting point for evaluations is the requirement to demonstrate value for money. These evaluations are typically quantitative, emphasising efficiency metrics and cost-benefit analysis. While this was not the main impetus behind the hospital AHPRC evaluation, elements of economic concern did surface—particularly in challenges related to sustaining the AHPRC under tight resource constraints.

Key stakeholders noted difficulties in releasing staff for practice development work due to budget limitations. This highlights the practical importance of including a value-for-money lens in even internally motivated evaluations. Future evaluations could incorporate baseline costing and performance indicators, a suggestion raised by staff as a missed opportunity during the initial implementation of the AHPRC.

Programme evaluation as a management requirement

Evaluations driven by management typically seek to understand whether a programme is operating efficiently and whether alternative delivery models could improve effectiveness. In the case study, these questions manifested in efforts to map the AHPRC's processes, establish performance indicators, and assess whether its structure delivered intended results.

Management-oriented concerns were addressed through qualitative inquiry into how the AHPRC operated day-to-day and whether staff were empowered by its structure. Staff were given input through democratic processes such as ballots and project selection, and their views were solicited via interviews. These procedural insights proved vital in understanding the strengths and limitations of the unit, including issues around communication and structural support.

Evaluation reflecting professional commitment to improvement

At the most internally driven end of the continuum lies a professional commitment to continuous quality improvement. This was arguably the core motivation behind the AHPRC evaluation. The programme itself was designed around principles of evidence-based practice, self-driven staff development, and interprofessional collaboration—hallmarks of a reflective, practitioner-led improvement model.

The evaluation adopted the Trident model, which explores outcomes, processes, and stakeholder perspectives. This alignment underscores how professional curiosity and accountability can guide a comprehensive, developmental evaluation. For instance, staff narratives revealed not just changes in patient care practices, but shifts in cultural norms—such as the move toward questioning traditional methods and embracing more evidence-based standards.

TRANSLATING STARTING POINTS INTO EVALUATION QUESTIONS

The chapter proposal articulates typical questions that arise from different starting points. The AHPRC case provides tangible examples of how these questions materialized:

- **Is the programme achieving its objectives?**
  Evaluation of outcomes was anchored in original goals set by the AHPRC—such as staff development, the introduction of care pathways, and improved patient care. Document review and stakeholder interviews revealed that many of these objectives were partially or fully achieved, although some, like formal research outputs, fell short.
- **Is the programme cost-effective and sustainable?**
  While this was not a central aim, challenges around funding and resource allocation were documented and used to recommend improvements in sustainability planning.
- **Is innovative practice working?**
  The evaluation identified tangible improvements in clinical care, staff morale, and recruitment, attributed to the AHPRC's influence. The emergence of new roles and the retention of a development-focused culture even after the AHPRC's formal end suggested successful innovation.
- **How can it be further developed?**
  Suggestions for improvement included introducing performance indicators from the outset, institutionalising the AHPRC model across the entire hospital, and enhancing the university's contribution.

METHODOLOGICAL TRANSLATION OF STARTING POINTS

Each starting point implies particular methodological choices. For instance, externally mandated evaluations often prioritise quantitative data and standardised metrics. By contrast, the AHPRC evaluation employed a qualitative methodology aligned with its internal, developmental purpose.

A thematic network analysis was used to distil rich, narrative data from interviews into organising and global themes. This method was particularly well-suited to exploring personal development, staff morale, and the subtleties of partnership dynamics—topics that resist easy quantification but are central to understanding programme impact in practice-based settings.

Moreover, sampling was conducted using an expanding method, beginning with key informants and growing organically—again reflecting the exploratory, insider-led nature of the evaluation. Ethical considerations were addressed through transparency, informed consent, and the appropriate setting of the project as a low-risk service evaluation.

STAKEHOLDER ENGAGEMENT: RESPONDING TO MULTIPLE PERSPECTIVES

Although the evaluation only formally included one group of stakeholders (staff directly involved in the AHPRC), the evaluation approach recognised the multiplicity of roles and experiences within this group. The evaluation thus preserved the spirit of the Trident model's commitment to pluralistic inquiry.

For future evaluations, particularly those situated at the midpoint or external end of the continuum, a broader stakeholder engagement strategy—including patients, community representatives, and institutional partners—would strengthen the evaluation's credibility and comprehensiveness.

INTEGRATING THE EVALUATION TRIDENT WITH STARTING POINTS

The Trident Evaluation Model, which examines outcomes, processes, and stakeholder perspectives, maps well onto the typology of starting points. Each prong can be selectively emphasised depending on the origin of the evaluation.

- **Outcomes** are especially pertinent to funding-driven evaluations and to managerial assessments of success.
- **Process** analysis is critical when internal learning and adaptation are central as was the case with the AHPRC.
- **Stakeholder perspectives** become essential in professional or developmental evaluations, where legitimacy and improvement are tightly tied to lived experience.

The AHPRC case shows how these elements can interrelate. For example, improved outcomes in recruitment and retention were explained through stakeholder insights about increased staff morale—thus connecting the "outcome" and "perspective" prongs. Similarly, the process of selecting projects through staff ballots reinforced the inclusive, developmental aims of the unit.

PRACTICAL IMPLICATIONS FOR EVALUATORS

By examining how the AHPRC evaluation aligned with different starting points, several practical lessons emerge for future evaluators:

1. **Clarify the Origin**
   Understanding the degrees of whether the evaluation is compliance-driven, management-led, or improvement-oriented will help tailor methods and expectations accordingly.
2. **Use Mixed Methods Thoughtfully**
   Qualitative methods offer depth in internally driven evaluations. However, incorporating baseline measures or performance indicators, even in qualitative studies, can strengthen accountability and future planning.
3. **Attend to Process and Culture**
   Evaluation should go beyond measuring outcomes to understand the processes and cultural dynamics that enable or inhibit success.
4. **Engage Stakeholders Early and Often**
   Especially when legitimacy and improvement are the goals, early stakeholder involvement enhances buy-in, enriches data, and fosters collective learning.
5. **Plan for Legacy**
   Evaluations should not only capture present outcomes but also consider the sustainability and diffusion of innovations, as evidenced by the enduring practice development culture in the case study.

CONCLUSION

Evaluation starting points shape every stage of the evaluation process—from design to analysis to use. Whether prompted by funders, managers, or professionals themselves, evaluations can benefit from a structured understanding of their origin and corresponding methodological fit. The case of the hospital AHPRC demonstrates how an internally motivated evaluation can successfully employ the Trident model to deliver actionable insights while fostering a culture of practice improvement. For evaluators, recognising and adapting to these starting points is not just a conceptual exercise—it is the foundation of meaningful, context-sensitive evaluation practice.

CHAPTER 5

Preliminary questions

Framing a programme evaluation of a community safety initiative with exploratory questions & considerations

INTRODUCTION

Before undertaking a programme evaluation, there are essential questions that must be addressed. These questions go beyond logistics or technical frameworks; they concern the underlying motivations, objectives, assumptions, and expectations that shape the evaluation's value and utility. Understanding why a programme is being evaluated—and what concerns might be anticipated—ensures that the evaluation process is meaningful, strategic, and ethically sound. This chapter provides a practical framework for addressing preliminary questions in programme evaluation, drawing upon the Trident model and lessons from a multi-agency safety initiative evaluated in a case study. The aim is to guide evaluators and programme leaders in clarifying their intentions, anticipating concerns, and establishing solid ground for an impactful evaluation.

WHY COMMISSION AN EVALUATION?

A programme evaluation is rarely a neutral exercise. It is often commissioned in response to evolving programme goals, funding pressures, political priorities, or stakeholder concerns. In the featured case study—a community safety initiative aimed at improving safety and information flow—evaluation was prompted by several converging factors. These included questions about the initiative's long-term viability, evolving initial objectives, overlapping agency responsibilities, and the need to assess whether community engagement had been meaningfully achieved.

DOI: 10.4324/9781003312253-5

Commissioning an evaluation in this context reflected a desire to take stock of what had been accomplished and to determine how best to adapt to a changing environment. Importantly, the programme had shifted from a single-agency initiative to a broader partnership model involving local governance, emergency services, and community volunteers. As such, the evaluation served not only to measure outcomes but to reassess purpose, effectiveness, and relevance.

This rationale applies broadly: evaluations should be commissioned when there is a need to confirm alignment between a programme's implementation and its intended objectives, particularly where resources, partnerships, and expectations are in flux. Evaluation also becomes vital when stakeholder confidence needs to be re-established, as was the case in this initiative where residents' familiarity with the programme varied significantly by locality.

In practical terms, a programme should be evaluated when:

- The objectives have evolved or are ambiguous.
- There is uncertainty about the programme's impact.
- Multiple stakeholders have divergent perspectives on what success looks like.
- There is pressure to demonstrate value-for-money or compliance with policy objectives.

CONCERNS TO ANTICIPATE

Any evaluation process carries potential concerns—some strategic, others ethical or operational. The most common concerns include:

- Fear that the evaluation will expose programme weaknesses.
- Worries about the fairness and accuracy of the evaluation process.
- Concerns that the findings might be misused or politically manipulated.
- Anxiety from staff or volunteers about the implications of performance.
- Ambiguity around what "success" really means for a complex programme.

In the case study, concerns included the limited engagement from community volunteers, which raised fears that the programme lacked legitimacy among its core constituents. There was also apprehension about whether the initiative's outcomes could be meaningfully assessed, given that many objectives were process-focused rather than outcome-based. Stakeholders were uneasy about whether the evaluation would appropriately reflect the subtleties of working in certain community contexts—where the perception of safety often mattered more than actual crime rates.

Such concerns underscore the importance of transparency and clarity in framing evaluations. Evaluators must work closely with commissioning agencies to define realistic expectations, set clear boundaries, and establish how findings will be interpreted and used.

CLARIFYING OUTCOMES: WHAT IS THE PROGRAMME TRYING TO ACHIEVE?

A foundational step in preparing for an evaluation is articulating the programme's intended outcomes. These should be stated clearly enough to guide assessment and flexible enough to reflect local realities. The Trident model encourages evaluators to ask: what are the expected outcomes? What indicators will show that these outcomes have been achieved?

In the case study, the initiative's early goals were somewhat vague and rooted in a general desire to reduce fear of crime and enhance community communication. Over time, as the project became integrated into a formal partnership model, its objectives became more specific: support for volunteers, expanded coordinator roles, acquisition of equipment, and public engagement. However, these remained predominantly process goals, focused on delivery mechanisms rather than measurable change.

For a robust evaluation, it is essential to move from process objectives to outcome objectives. Instead of asking whether a public safety leaflet was distributed, evaluators should ask: did recipients report greater knowledge of safety practices? Did perceptions of safety improve in areas where interventions occurred?

The evaluative questions that follow from this include:

- What were the intended short- and long-term effects?
- Were there quantifiable indicators tied to these effects?
- What baseline data exists to support before-and-after comparisons?
- How will qualitative evidence (e.g., stakeholder testimonies) be integrated?

Clarifying these points before the evaluation begins ensures that the evaluation is measuring the right things and that the programme's vision of success is coherent.

UNDERSTANDING PROCESS: HOW IS THE PROGRAMME IMPLEMENTED?

Once outcomes are defined, the next set of preliminary questions involves the programme's process. These include:

- How is the programme structured?
- Are the implementation methods clearly specified?
- Can the programme be replicated elsewhere?
- What are the innovations introduced and how do they differ from previous efforts?

In this case, process mapping revealed a top-down communication structure. Information typically flowed from statutory agencies through a coordinator to community volunteers. Feedback mechanisms existed but were under-utilised. The process evaluation showed how implementation structure, staff roles, and volunteer management shaped the programme's functioning.

A key insight was the importance of the coordinator role in bridging institutional frameworks with community needs. However, limited hours, varied volunteer training, and weak bidirectional communication created gaps. While some residents had never heard of the initiative; others saw the initiative as essential.

Evaluators should gather evidence such as meeting minutes, communication logs, operational manuals, and observations of staff practice. The goal is to understand whether the programme is being delivered as intended—and whether the delivery model itself is fit for purpose. In the example, innovations such as a structured community walk with police officers offered opportunities for community engagement, but the uneven take-up highlighted process weaknesses.

Another consideration is resource allocation. Are costs in line with comparable interventions? Does the programme offer value relative to its scale and reach? In the case study, the programme consumed a disproportionate share of safety funding, raising questions about strategic resource deployment.

STAKEHOLDERS: WHOSE VOICES COUNT?

Stakeholders form the third prong of the Trident model. Any evaluation must address whose perspectives are relevant and how these will be captured. The preliminary questions here include:

- Who are the key stakeholders?
- What roles do they play in programme design, delivery, or use?
- What are their expectations, interests, and concerns?

This case study offered a rich set of stakeholder perspectives—statutory agencies, community volunteers, Steering Group members, and residents. Each held different assumptions about the purpose of the initiative. Some stakeholders believed the project was about crime reduction, while others saw it as addressing broader quality-of-life issues such as traffic safety, noise, or intergenerational tension.

Capturing this plurality requires deliberate design. In the evaluation, surveys, focus groups, and interviews were used to gather data. However, participation varied: residents were relatively responsive; volunteers, less so. This discrepancy raised concerns about how representative the evaluation findings were—an issue any evaluator must anticipate.

Evaluators should also be prepared to handle conflicting accounts. For example, while officials viewed certain resources used in the programme as important assets, volunteers were less convinced of their utility—possibly due to maintenance issues unknown to decision-makers. Such differences illustrate why triangulating data from multiple stakeholders is essential for a balanced evaluation.

Framing baselines and comparative evidence

Evaluation requires comparison. Yet meaningful comparisons rely on establishing baseline data. Before launching the evaluation do consider:

- What pre-existing data are available?
- How reliable are these sources?
- Are there historic trends or previous evaluations to draw upon?

In this initiative the baseline was limited. Early phases of the initiative were not well documented and performance metrics were poorly defined. Later objectives remained too process-oriented to support comparative analysis. The evaluation addressed this gap by triangulating survey data, resident feedback, and crime statistics.

Establishing a credible baseline can be challenging, particularly when programs evolve rapidly or operate in dynamic environments. Nevertheless, efforts should be made to document initial conditions, ideally including:

- Community needs assessments.
- Crime or safety statistics.
- Historical programme funding and staffing levels.
- Qualitative accounts of public perceptions.

These data points allow for a more nuanced understanding of change and help determine whether observed impacts are attributable to the programme itself.

MANAGING ETHICAL AND PRACTICAL RISKS

Commissioners and evaluators must also consider practical and ethical challenges. These include:

- Maintaining confidentiality and informed consent.
- Avoiding conflict of interest, particularly in stakeholder-led evaluations.
- Ensuring transparency in data interpretation.
- Balancing critique with constructive feedback.

This case study highlighted a tension between the need for honest feedback and the desire to protect the goodwill of community volunteers. Some volunteers expressed frustration with how the programme was managed while others were disengaged. Ethical evaluation practice involves listening without blame and making space for divergent perspectives.

Moreover, when evaluations are used to justify continued funding, there is a risk that findings may be distorted or overly optimistic. Commissioners should clarify at the outset how findings will be used and whether they are intended to support funding applications, strategic planning, or public accountability.

PREPARING FOR EVALUATION: A CHECKLIST

Drawing on the issues explored above, the following checklist may assist programme leaders and evaluators in preparing for a rigorous, useful evaluation:

1. **Purpose**: Clearly articulate why the evaluation is being conducted. Is it for learning, accountability, redesign, or funding?
2. **Outcomes**: Define intended outcomes in specific, measurable terms. Include both process and impact goals.
3. **Processes**: Document how the programme operates. Include staffing structures, delivery mechanisms, innovations, and logistics.
4. **Stakeholders**: Identify who needs to be involved. Plan for inclusive and representative engagement.
5. **Baseline Data**: Gather existing evidence or develop methods for retrospective baseline construction.
6. **Risks and Concerns**: Anticipate ethical issues, stakeholder fears, and operational constraints. Build mitigation strategies.
7. **Evaluation Questions**: Frame clear, aligned evaluation questions across the Trident dimensions (outcomes, processes, stakeholder perspectives).
8. **Use of Findings**: Decide how the evaluation results will be disseminated and applied.

CONCLUSION

Preliminary exploratory questions may seem basic but they form the foundation of effective programme evaluation. Clarifying why a programme is being evaluated and anticipating associated concerns, is not just good planning—it is ethical, strategic, and essential to achieving meaningful insight.

The case study of this initiative illustrates the complexity of programme intentions, stakeholder dynamics, and implementation realities. By addressing preliminary questions through the Trident lens, programme leaders and evaluators can develop evaluations that are not only methodologically sound but also deeply relevant to the communities and systems they seek to support and improve.

APPENDIX: PRELIMINARY QUESTIONNAIRE TOOL

Before starting an evaluation, we ask the evaluation initiators to consider a number of questions to clarify their expectations and better prepare for the evaluation itself. Their responses make a good starting point for the partnership planning of the evaluation through the Steering Group (see below).

SUPPORTING THE DESIGN OF A PROGRAMME EVALUATION

Thank you for considering support or sponsorship of a programme evaluation. To help us tailor an effective and relevant evaluation plan, we kindly ask for your responses to the following questions. These are grouped into key areas: **Expectations, Outcomes, Processes,** and **Stakeholder Perspectives.**

Please answer as fully as possible. Your responses will help shape the scope, design, and utility of the evaluation for all involved parties.

1. **Expectations**

    - What are your primary reasons for supporting or sponsoring this evaluation?
      (e.g., strategic insight, accountability, funding justification, learning)
    - What are your key expectations or goals for what the evaluation should deliver?
      (e.g., outcome data, process review, return on investment, policy recommendations)
    - Are there specific questions or themes you would like the evaluation to address?
    - Do you have any concerns or reservations about the evaluation?
      (e.g., timescale, access to data, risk to reputation, stakeholder sensitivities)

2. **Outcomes**

    - What are the main outcomes or impacts the programme is intended to achieve?
      (List short-, medium-, and long-term intended changes if possible)
    - By which specific outcomes should the programme be judged?
    - What kinds of evidence do you expect will demonstrate these outcomes?
      (e.g., quantitative performance data, user feedback, qualitative accounts)
    - Is there existing baseline or comparative data against which to assess change?
      (e.g., previous programme performance, community indicators, historical trends)

3. **Processes**

    - Are there clear specifications or models for how the programme is delivered?
      (e.g., guidelines, service standards, staffing models, protocols)
    - Could the current programme structure be replicated elsewhere with the existing documentation?
    - What lessons have been learned from the programme's delivery to date?
    - How do current programme costs compare with prior or similar provision?
    - What are the most distinctive or innovative aspects of the programme?
      (e.g., unique partnerships, digital tools, culturally specific approaches)
    - How many service users are expected to participate during the evaluation period?

4. **Stakeholder Perspectives**

- Who are the key stakeholders that the evaluation should consider?
  (e.g., service users, programme staff, delivery partners, community members, policymakers)
- Are there particular stakeholder groups whose feedback should be prioritised?
  (e.g., funders, marginalised groups, frontline workers)
- Are there any stakeholders whose support or insight is crucial to programme success or sustainability?

Please return your responses to the evaluation team. Your input ensures the evaluation will be strategically aligned, focused on real-world impact, and beneficial for current and future funding decisions and participant experience.

CHAPTER 6

The Steering Group and partnership

How to build effective partnerships between evaluators and programme stakeholders in programme evaluation

We have found the most effective way to conduct a programme evaluation is on the basis of a developing a partnership between the evaluators and those who are delivering, supporting and engaging in the programme. The cooperation of the providers is essential in order to give access to the data required to address the evaluation questions. And, in many cases, the providers themselves may be gathering these data as part of a routine with regard to agreed outcomes or surveying perspectives. And, of course, this also builds a cohesive group that is primarily focused on the evaluation itself which is valuable to the evaluators for a number of reasons including establishing a shared mission for the evaluation with agreed questions and data to be gathered to address them. The Steering Group is both a sounding board for ideas and approaches and also the formal recipient of plans and reports.

The Steering Group partners should agree the purpose and approach of the evaluation and recognise that the interim reports and the final report will publicise the successful features of the programme and will also provide feedback for a process of Continuous Quality Improvement.

The partnership is reflected in a Steering Group which will be made up of the evaluators, the providers or programme deliverers, together with representatives of programme participants (if possible) and funders. An example of Steering Group membership and terms of reference are as follows:

SOCIAL HEALTH AND EVALUATION UNIT

Programme evaluation Steering Groups

At the beginning of a programme evaluation, an Evaluation Steering Group will be established consisting of the evaluators and representatives nominated by the contractor.

DOI: 10.4324/9781003312253-6

The Steering Group will be in existence for the life of the evaluation. The Steering Group will meet on an agreed schedule but at the very least twice, once at the beginning of the evaluation and once at the end. The Steering Group is likely to be chaired by the senior member of the evaluation team. It will be supported in note taking and arrangements by either an administrator from the contracting group or a member of the evaluation team

The terms of reference for the Steering Group will include the following.

- To agree the overall design of the evaluation and the mini-projects which will make up the evaluation.
- To facilitate access for the evaluators to data concerning the programme.
- To receive reports from the evaluators.
- To agree the publication and dissemination of findings.
- To promote the implementation of the recommendations.

ESTABLISHING AND BUILDING EVALUATION PARTNERSHIPS IN A CASE STUDY

Introduction

Effective programme evaluation hinges not only on methodological rigour but also on the strength of relationships between evaluators and those delivering and receiving the programme. This chapter explores how to cultivate and sustain partnerships between evaluators and stakeholders—including funders, providers, and service users—using practical guidance grounded in applied experience. Drawing on anonymised case material from a mental health collaborative, this chapter provides actionable advice for building meaningful evaluation partnerships that foster trust, improve data quality, and promote shared learning.

At the heart of this chapter, is the concept of partnership-based evaluation, where the process is jointly owned and shaped by both evaluators and participants. It outlines the key principles that underpin successful evaluator *programme relationships* and highlights mechanisms such as Evaluation Steering Groups and discusses practical tools for assessing partnership dynamics. By following these steps, evaluators can move beyond detached observation to become embedded collaborators who add value throughout the evaluation cycle.

UNDERSTANDING EVALUATION AS A PARTNERSHIP

Moving beyond external scrutiny

Traditional models of evaluation often position the evaluator as an external observer tasked with judging programme effectiveness. While independent scrutiny remains important, contemporary practice increasingly recognises that collaborative models can yield richer insights and more sustainable improvements. When evaluators engage as partners rather than external auditors, they better understand contextual knowledge and operational realities that would otherwise remain hidden.

In this case material, evaluators embedded within a managed health collaborative were able to co-develop evaluation tools and priorities with programme staff. This partnership led to the adaptation of a national assessment framework to include local demographics, five-point Likert scales, and qualitative data. The modifications enhanced relevance, increased staff engagement, and ensured the findings were meaningful to those most affected.

Shared ownership of evaluation questions

The foundation of any successful evaluation partnership is shared agreement on what the evaluation seeks to understand. Evaluation questions should be co-designed by evaluators and stakeholders, including funders, programme managers, front-line staff, and where appropriate, service users. This co-creation ensures that the evaluation speaks to real-world concerns and builds mutual investment in its outcomes.

In practice, this means convening planning meetings early in the process to develop agreed-upon evaluation aims. In one case, the evaluation team worked with leadership and practitioners to identify key themes around integration, communication, and user outcomes. This consensus enabled the evaluation to focus not only on service metrics but also on the intangible dynamics of cross-agency collaboration.

MECHANISMS FOR SUPPORTING PARTNERSHIP: THE ROLE OF EVALUATION STEERING GROUPS

Composition and purpose

Evaluation Steering Groups (ESGs) provide an institutional mechanism to maintain partnership throughout the evaluation lifecycle. Typically composed of evaluators, programme deliverers, funders, and sometimes recipient representatives, these groups meet regularly to guide evaluation design, monitor progress, troubleshoot challenges, assist in facilitating work, and interpret findings.

In this particular case material, the ESG played a pivotal role in aligning the evaluation with local priorities. It served as a forum for diverse views, allowing members to surface differing expectations and clarify roles. Importantly, the ESG structure created a space where concerns could be addressed collaboratively, reducing tensions and improving the quality of data provided.

Managing power dynamics

One challenge in forming effective ESGs is navigating the inherent power imbalances between evaluators, funders, and delivery agents. Transparency about purpose, roles, and influence is essential. Clear terms of reference can help delineate responsibilities and decision-making protocols, ensuring that all voices are heard.

In one example, therapists within the collaborative initially felt marginalised in the evaluation planning. However, following with their integration into the ESG, their perspectives were able to shape the design of the partnership assessment tools, leading to a more meaningful and balanced measure of collaboration. This inclusivity increased trust and generated richer qualitative insights during the data collection phase and throughout the evaluation cycle.

SUPPORTING COLLABORATIVE DATA GENERATION

Agreement on data streams and sources

Effective partnership requires alignment on what data will be collected, how, and for what purpose. Evaluators should not simply impose data requirements but should instead work with stakeholders to *identify feasible and meaningful data streams.* These may include quantitative service metrics, staff surveys, focus groups, and administrative records.

In this case material, the evaluation team adapted a pre-existing partnership tool in dialogue with local staff. Modifications included demographic variables tailored to the service, a five-point Likert scale, and open-ended questions. This collaborative design ensured the instrument captured not only standardised metrics but also contextual insights valued by programme staff.

Ensuring validity through participatory engagement

Partnership-based evaluation does not compromise methodological rigour; rather, it enhances it by drawing on firsthand knowledge. Staff can identify confounding variables, suggest alternative interpretations of data, and validate emerging findings. Their participation also increases the likelihood that the findings will be implemented.

For example, front-line practitioners helped interpret mixed findings about trust within the collaborative. While quantitative data suggested high trust levels, qualitative responses revealed persistent tensions between statutory and voluntary sector partners. Joint analysis workshops helped surface these discrepancies and identify actionable steps for improvement, such as, facilitated team-building sessions.

DEVELOPING AND SHARING RECOMMENDATIONS

Co-producing recommendations

Evaluation findings must be translated into recommendations that are actionable, context-sensitive, and acceptable to those who will implement them. This process benefits from joint analysis and co-authorship. Evaluators can present preliminary findings to ESGs or broader stakeholder groups to test interpretations and refine proposals.

In the case material, evaluators facilitated reflection sessions where programme staff reviewed the partnership tool findings and collaboratively developed improvement plans. For example, the need to clarify discharge pathways and service outcomes emerged from staff feedback, not evaluator imposition. These co-produced recommendations carried greater legitimacy and were more likely to be achieved.

Feeding findings back into organisational learning

One advantage of a partnership model is that learning can occur throughout the evaluation, not just at the end. Interim feedback loops—such as progress reports, learning seminars, or reflective team meetings—allow organisations to adjust practice in real time.

In a follow-up assessment, many staff commented positively on the collaboratives' responsiveness to earlier evaluation findings. Improvements in communication processes and clearer role definitions had been implemented based on previous evaluation rounds. This feedback loop illustrates how *partnership evaluation fosters learning, continuous quality improvement and organisational evolution.*

ASSESSING THE QUALITY OF PARTNERSHIP

Using structured tools

To maintain strong evaluator–programme relationships, it is helpful to periodically assess the quality of the partnership itself. Tools such as a communication or partnership audits can offer structured methods to explore areas for clarity of purpose, trust, ownership, and communication.

In the case material, the partnership tool provided a snapshot of how staff experienced partnership working across six core principles. While overall feedback was positive, some areas—such as equitable resource contribution and communication across dispersed teams—were flagged for improvement. This feedback allowed targeted interventions, such as improved information-sharing protocols and training on partnership working.

Interpreting discrepant data

Quantitative assessments can sometimes mask underlying tensions. For example, high average scores on trust might obscure divergent views between different staff groups. Therefore, it is critical to combine survey data with qualitative insights and to explore contradictions rather than gloss over them.

In the case material, qualitative responses revealed lingering concerns among some staff about multi-agency integration and identity preservation. By explicitly addressing these in feedback sessions, evaluators helped the programme navigate sensitive terrain without undermining overall cohesion.

SUSTAINING PARTNERSHIP THROUGH ORGANISATIONAL CHANGE

Partnerships are dynamic

Organisations evolve and so do evaluation partnerships. Staff turnover, funding changes, and shifting policy landscapes can affect partnership dynamics. Evaluators need to anticipate and manage these transitions, ensuring that new participants are oriented to the shared evaluation approach.

In this instance, several respondents noted that changes in senior leadership had both positive and negative impacts on the partnership. Maintaining continuity through documentation, role clarity, and mentoring helped preserve the evaluation ethos across personnel changes.

Embedding evaluation capacity

One legacy of strong evaluation partnerships is *enhanced internal capacity for reflective practice*. When staff participate meaningfully in evaluation, they acquire skills and confidence to undertake future evaluations themselves. Building this capacity may involve mentoring, training, or co-analysis activities during the evaluation.

This evaluation work contributed to internal development. Staff reported improved understanding of evaluation concepts, greater willingness to engage with data, and increased ownership of service improvement efforts. These outcomes reflect the long-term value of investing in evaluator–programme relationships.

CONCLUSION: KEY LESSONS FOR PRACTICE

Evaluation partnerships thrive on trust, mutual respect, and shared purpose. The case examples discussed illustrate that when evaluators and programme stakeholders collaborate throughout the evaluation process—from question development to data analysis to dissemination—findings are more credible, relevant, and actionable. To achieve this, evaluators should:

- Engage stakeholders early and often.
- Establish inclusive structures such as ESGs.
- Co-create data tools and evaluation questions.
- Facilitate joint interpretation of findings.
- Embed opportunities for real-time feedback and learning.
- Use structured tools to monitor the partnership itself.

Most importantly, evaluators must recognise that relationships are not peripheral to evaluation—they are central to its success. By adopting a Partnership Approach, evaluators become *enablers of organisational learning and co-creators of change*.

CHAPTER 7

Evaluation questions and data streams

Structuring inquiry through the Trident Evaluation Model

INTRODUCTION: ANCHORING EVALUATION IN STRATEGIC QUESTIONS

At the core of any meaningful programme evaluation lies the formulation of carefully structured questions and the systematic collection of relevant data. These are not simply operational necessities; they serve as the architecture upon which all analysis, interpretation, and ultimately, policy or practice recommendations rest. Without focused and relevant evaluation questions, data collection becomes diffuse and interpretation arbitrary.

The ***Trident Evaluation Model***, with its three-pronged structure—*outcomes, processes, and stakeholder perspectives*—offers a strategic approach to question development. By considering each dimension in tandem and interaction, evaluators are better equipped to navigate complexity, uncover mechanisms, and ensure the evaluation remains grounded in the programme's practical realities.

This chapter provides guidance on how to generate evaluation questions and corresponding data strategies using the Trident model. Drawing on an anonymised case study of a public energy efficiency initiative—focused on community centres—the chapter shows how theoretical structures can be translated into applied evaluation logic.

THE ROLE OF THE TRIDENT MODEL IN FRAMING EVALUATION LOGIC

The Trident model serves as both a *theoretical anchor and a practical tool*. Each of its three elements represents a different line of inquiry, yet all intersect and inform one another. Structuring an evaluation with this model ensures that evaluators do not overly privilege technical outcomes while neglecting implementation processes or human engagement—an imbalance common in narrowly scoped evaluations.

DOI: 10.4324/9781003312253-7

In practice, this means evaluators begin by identifying key questions under each prong, while recognising that answers in one domain may shape findings in another. The community centre case study demonstrates how this model can guide evaluations even in decentralised, volunteer-led, and resource-constrained contexts.

OUTCOMES: WHAT CHANGED AND WHY IT MATTERS

Framing outcome questions

Outcome questions are designed to assess the *effectiveness and impact* of a programme. These may be defined in terms of behavioural change, material improvement, cost savings, environmental effects, or shifts in social awareness. Effective outcome questions are *specific, measurable, and meaningfully aligned with programme objectives.*

In the community centre evaluation, outcome-related questions included:

- To what extent did energy consumption decrease following retrofitting?
- How did building characteristics affect the efficacy of energy-saving measures?
- Were there observable shifts in environmental awareness or practice among hall committees?

These questions linked measurable changes (e.g., kWh reduction) with interpretive elements (e.g., sustainability awareness), making space for both quantitative and qualitative insights.

Data streams

To answer these questions, the evaluators combined:

- Longitudinal energy use data (before and after upgrades).
- Building profiles (age, size, insulation type).
- Cost records (heating bills, retrofit investment).
- Stakeholder reflections (on perceived effectiveness and motivation).

Findings showed that halls with comprehensive insulation and modern heating saw the greatest energy savings. However, symbolic or educational outcomes—such as use of the building as a community exemplar—were inconsistently realised, indicating that technical improvements alone were insufficient for broader impact.

Practical implications

A narrow focus on immediate consumption metrics would have missed the longer-term, community-level significance of the halls as sustainability demonstrators. Hence, outcome evaluations must ***expand beyond cost-benefit frames*** to include symbolic, institutional, and social dimensions.

PROCESS: UNDERSTANDING HOW DELIVERY SHAPES RESULTS

Framing process questions

Process evaluation focuses on the *means by which outcomes are achieved*—and where they are hindered. These questions consider logistics, sequencing, coordination, and resource access. They are especially important in multi-actor or community-driven projects where variability in delivery can heavily influence performance.

Relevant questions from the case study included:

- What practical steps were required to access and implement energy-saving measures?
- How did funding mechanisms shape the scope of building improvements?
- What challenges did committees face in managing installation and maintenance?

Data streams

Here, data included:

- Completed questionnaires describing renovation actions and timelines.
- Qualitative interviews on difficulties in navigating funding or technical guidance.
- Documentation on grant application processes and available support materials.

These data revealed considerable *fragmentation and inefficiency*. Projects were often driven by opportunistic, one-off funding bids rather than long-term energy strategies. For example, one hall installed a modern heating system without first insulating the space, resulting in minimal energy savings and extended return on investment.

Many committees reported challenges in identifying suitable contractors, lack of clarity in available guidance, and poor coordination between funding schemes. As a result, implementation was uneven, and full potential gains were unrealised.

Practical implications

Without well-resourced and integrated implementation pathways, even well-conceived programs falter. Process evaluations can diagnose these weaknesses and highlight necessary improvements in institutional design, communication, and capacity-building.

STAKEHOLDER PERSPECTIVES: WHO IS INVOLVED, AND HOW DO THEY PERCEIVE THE PROGRAMME?

Framing perspective questions

The third Trident prong examines how *different actors experience and interpret the programme*. This includes exploring variation in values, priorities, understandings, and expectations. Particularly in community settings, stakeholder perspectives shape not only participation but also sustainability.

Key questions from the case study included:

- How do committee members define their role regarding environmental responsibility?
- What attitudes exist toward sustainability and energy-saving investments?
- How do hall users (e.g., community groups) interact with or affect building energy usage?

Data streams

Evaluators used:

- Semi-structured interviews with committee members.
- Questionnaires capturing levels of engagement and motivation.
- Observations about hall use patterns and scheduling.

The findings revealed a *narrow view of committee responsibility*—typically confined to basic hall maintenance and user bookings. Few saw themselves as environmental stewards. This constrained ambition and discouraged proactive planning.

Even where sustainability was acknowledged as important, limited confidence, technical knowledge, and support led to inertia. Further, varying energy expectations among user groups (e.g., exercise classes vs. senior meetings) complicated thermal management.

Practical implications

Evaluating stakeholder perspectives clarifies where *capacity-building and narrative shifts* are needed. It also reminds evaluators that sustainable infrastructure change requires alignment between values, responsibilities, and institutional context.

INTEGRATING THE PRONGS: BUILDING A COHERENT EVALUATION STRATEGY

The *true strength of the Trident model* lies in its integrative logic. Outcome results are shaped by implementation processes, which in turn are influenced by stakeholder beliefs and capacities. Evaluators should look for *feedback loops and causal relationships*, not just parallel categories.

For instance:

- Weak energy savings (outcome) were often due to incomplete retrofits (process), which were a result of limited committee ambition or knowledge (stakeholder perspective).
- In halls where committees viewed sustainability as part of their leadership role (perspective), implementation was more systematic (process), and energy use fell (outcome).

This integrative approach allows evaluations to go beyond *what worked*, and explore *why*, *for whom*, and *under what conditions*—questions that ultimately make findings actionable.

OPERATIONALISING THE TRIDENT IN PRACTICE: TOOLS AND TEMPLATES

To support practical use of this model, evaluators may wish to develop:

- An *evaluation matrix*, mapping questions across each Trident prong with linked data sources.
- A *data collection schedule*, ensuring timing aligns with key implementation phases.
- A *participatory design process*, co-developing questions with key stakeholders to enhance relevance and buy-in.
- A *reflexive review cycle*, adapting questions and tools as the evaluation progresses.

These practices help maintain rigour while remaining responsive to evolving programme dynamics.

CONCLUSION: DESIGNING EVALUATIONS THAT REFLECT REAL-*WORLD* COMPLEXITY

Using the Trident model to structure evaluation questions and data streams enables evaluators to capture the *complex, interactive nature of real-world programs.* The community centre case study illustrates that energy efficiency outcomes are not simply technical matters, but socially and institutionally embedded challenges. Evaluations must reflect this overall dynamic and context.

By asking outcomes, processes, and stakeholder-oriented questions in concert—and linking them to appropriate data sources—evaluators produce findings that are not only accurate but actionable. In resource-constrained settings, this capacity to diagnose, explain, and guide improvement is especially valuable.

Ultimately, evaluation questions are the *strategic lens* through which a programme is interpreted. The Trident model ensures that this lens is wide enough to capture complexity but structured enough to produce clarity.

CHAPTER 8

Overall design and structure

The Evaluation Trident and connections

The Trident is a coherent way of organising evaluation questions. However, it is the connection between the prongs of the Trident which address many important questions. What is it in the process which brings about the important outcomes? For example, how do Physiotherapy exercises affect mobility or alleviate pain? In the classroom, what teaching methods lead to learning? Thus, it is important from the start to identify questions which concern and highlight connections between data streams.

In the evaluation of a service innovation, it is essential to identify what works and this needs outcomes to be related to process variables even though they are measured separately and possibly differently methodologically on the quantitative and qualitative spectrum.

The evaluation Trident data streams allow comparisons and contrasts to be made between the relatively objective data and outcomes and process and the more subjective impressions captured in multiple stakeholder perspectives.

The comparison between relatively external measurement in outcomes and process and the subjective impressions captured in multiple stakeholder perspectives gives an important dimension to the evaluation.

The Steering Group should consider the connections or hypotheses relating variables which the evaluation will address. It is usually the relationship between process and outcomes that the evaluation should explore and these should be expressed in a way that the data in the process stream and the outcome stream should allow for connections to be explored.

CONDUCTING A PROGRAMME EVALUATION USING THE TRIDENT MODEL: A CASE STUDY WITH A NEIGHBOURHOOD SAFETY HUB (NSH)

Introduction

Programme evaluation is a vital process in ensuring that public initiatives achieve their intended goals and deliver value to the communities they serve. Traditional

DOI: 10.4324/9781003312253-8

evaluation approaches often focus narrowly on outcomes, leaving gaps in understanding how a programme was implemented or how it was experienced by those involved. The Trident Evaluation Model addresses this limitation by offering a three-pronged framework that evaluates outcomes, processes, and stakeholder perspectives in an integrated way. It allows evaluators to ask not only whether a programme works, but how it works and for whom.

This guide provides a practical walkthrough of how to use the Trident model in programme evaluation. To ground the guidance in a real-world scenario, it draws on an anonymised case study of a Neighbourhood Safety Hub (NSH) that was designed to reduce anti-social behaviour and enhance inter-agency collaboration in a mid-sized urban area. The case offers rich insights into the challenges and successes of multi-agency community programs and illustrates how the Trident framework can provide a comprehensive evaluation.

Understanding the Trident model

The Trident Evaluation Model centers around three mutually reinforcing components: outcomes, processes, and stakeholder perspectives. Outcomes refer to the measurable changes that occur as a result of the programme. These might include shifts in crime rates, improvements in public safety, or increased efficiency in service delivery. The process component concerns how the programme was delivered, including the coordination among agencies, the design of service pathways, and the overall implementation. Stakeholder perspectives involve the experiences, perceptions, and insights of those involved in or affected by the programme, including staff, participants, partner organizations, and community members.

Crucially, these three components do not operate in isolation. Instead, they intersect to form a fuller picture of programme functioning. For instance, a programme may yield positive outcomes but be perceived negatively by service users if, for example, communication was poor. Alternatively, a well-received programme may fail to meet its intended goals due to operational inefficiencies. The Trident model encourages evaluators to examine these interactions in detail, producing evaluations that are both methodologically rigorous and contextually meaningful.

Step one: Defining the purpose of the evaluation

The first step in any evaluation is to clearly define its purpose. This foundational step influences the choice of methods, the framing of research questions, and the interpretation of findings. Evaluations can be formative, supporting the development or improvement of a programme; summative, assessing its effectiveness; or developmental, informing programs that are still evolving.

In the case of the NSH, the evaluation was both formative and summative. It aimed to assess the early impact of the centre on crime prevention, examine how inter-agency collaboration had improved since co-location, and understand how the centre was being perceived and used by the public. This multi-faceted purpose made the Trident model especially suitable, as it could address short-term achievements, operational processes, and community engagement in parallel.

Step two: Developing a theory of change

Developing a theory of change or logic model helps map out the programme's assumptions and causal pathways. This typically involves identifying the resources invested in the programme (such as staff, funding, and facilities), the activities undertaken (such as educational seminars or CCTV monitoring), and the outputs and outcomes expected. A well-articulated theory of change clarifies how change is anticipated to occur and provides a blueprint for evaluation.

For the NSH, the theory of change was based on several assumptions: that co-locating agencies would improve information sharing and coordination, that visible public safety infrastructure would reduce fear of crime, and that educational initiatives would increase community engagement in crime prevention. This model also included intermediate outcomes, such as improved communication between police and social services, which were expected to contribute to longer-term goals like reductions in anti-social behaviour and increased public trust in local institutions.

Step three: Designing the evaluation strategy

A robust evaluation strategy considers how to explore each of the three prongs of the Trident model using appropriate data sources and methods. For outcomes, evaluators gathered quantitative data on crime rates, incident reports, and usage statistics related to NSH services. These data were complemented by qualitative indicators, such as community members' feelings of safety and staff reflections on case resolution.

The process evaluation involved examining the NSH's physical layout, operating hours, inter-agency workflows, and service coordination mechanisms. Observational fieldwork, internal documents, and staff interviews were used to identify implementation challenges and successes.

To understand stakeholder perspectives, evaluators conducted semi-structured interviews and focus groups with diverse groups, including local residents, business owners, agency staff, and voluntary sector partners. These conversations revealed how the centre was viewed in terms of accessibility, responsiveness, and overall value.

By weaving these methods together, evaluators could produce a comprehensive assessment that went beyond a simple "success or failure" dichotomy and instead illuminated the nuanced ways in which the programme operated and was received.

Step four: Collecting and analysing data

Data collection in the Trident framework is inherently multi-method and iterative. In the NSH case study, quantitative data such as police statistics and service usage logs were analysed to detect patterns before and after the centre's implementation. These patterns were interpreted with caution, recognising that many factors can influence crime trends.

Qualitative data collection provided richer context. Observations at the NSH revealed how space was used and where bottlenecks occurred. For instance, it was noted that public access to the centre was limited during peak hours, undermining one of the core goals of enhancing community engagement. Interviews with staff exposed differing levels of buy-in, with some agencies more committed to the partnership than others.

Stakeholder interviews added a crucial dimension. Community members praised the concept of the NSH but often expressed uncertainty about what services were available. Some felt that the centre was not sufficiently advertised or physically visible. These perceptions helped explain why usage data was lower than expected, despite improvements in service coordination.

By triangulating across data sources, the evaluators could identify consistencies and contradictions, generating a more robust understanding of how the centre was functioning.

Step five: Interpreting findings across the three prongs

The interpretive phase involved synthesising data across the three dimensions. Positive outcomes, such as a plateau in crime rates and reduced emergency response times, were linked to improvements in inter-agency coordination. However, the evaluation also highlighted limitations in public outreach and visibility, which affected the NSH's ability to serve as a central hub for community engagement.

Process findings showed that while co-location facilitated faster decision-making among professionals, differences in agency cultures sometimes led to miscommunication. For example, staff from policing, youth work, and housing agencies brought different assumptions and procedures to joint meetings, requiring time and effort to harmonize.

From a stakeholder perspective, the centre's existence was broadly welcomed, but its impact was unevenly felt. Tourists and business owners noticed a more visible police presence and quicker responses to minor incidents, but some marginalised community members reported little change in their access to services or perception of safety.

These insights allowed evaluators to formulate recommendations that were both systemic and specific, addressing structural issues without losing sight of individual experiences.

Step six: Making evidence-based recommendations

The final report included recommendations across all three dimensions. To improve outcomes, the evaluators suggested extending service hours to better align with the night-time economy and increasing data collection on public perceptions of safety. In terms of process improvements, they advised adopting flexible workspace models (such as hot-desking) to allow for greater agency participation and installing safety measures for frontline staff, including a panic button system.

For stakeholder engagement, the evaluation emphasised the importance of a sustained communication strategy. This included rebranding the NSH, relocating signage for greater visibility, and holding regular public forums to update residents on services and invite feedback. Additionally, community groups were encouraged to participate in shaping service delivery, reinforcing the idea that safety is a shared responsibility.

Crucially, the recommendations were interlinked. Improved visibility would not only enhance stakeholder engagement but also help boost outcome metrics by encouraging higher service uptake. Streamlined workflows would support more consistent service delivery, improving user satisfaction and internal morale. This integrative approach is a hallmark of the Trident model and one of its core strengths.

Reflections on the Trident model in practice

The Trident model proved particularly effective for evaluating a complex initiative like the NSH, where multiple agencies, outcomes, and the public intersect. Its strength lies in its capacity to hold complexity without losing clarity, allowing evaluators to examine not just whether a programme worked, but how and why it did.

At the same time, the model is resource-intensive. Conducting a truly integrated evaluation requires time, diverse skillsets, and stakeholder cooperation. Conflicting data can also pose interpretive challenges. For instance, quantitative indicators might show improvement while qualitative feedback remains negative, necessitating careful reflection and transparent communication of findings.

Nonetheless, the model's comprehensiveness pays dividends. By examining implementation quality and lived experiences alongside outcome data, evaluators can provide a more honest and useful account of a programme's performance. In the NSH case, this led to a richer understanding of what made the centre work—and what needed refinement to better serve its community.

Conclusion

The NSH case study demonstrates how the Trident model can guide evaluations of multi-agency, public-facing initiatives. It shows the importance of integrating multiple viewpoints, measuring both tangible and intangible effects and remaining responsive to the evolving needs of stakeholders. For anyone undertaking a programme evaluation in today's dynamic social environment, the Trident model provides both structure and flexibility—two qualities essential to responsible and effective evaluation practice.

It is also important to see how programme evaluation is both a technical and ethical task, requiring methods that are robust, inclusive, and adaptable to real-world complexity. The Trident Evaluation Model offers a powerful framework for achieving this task. By systematically examining outcomes, processes, and stakeholder perspectives, evaluators can produce findings that are not only accurate but also meaningful and actionable.

CHAPTER 9

Project management and responsibilities

A practical guide to structuring and delivering effective evaluations with a case study of a community partnership service

Obviously, programs vary greatly in scale from; for example, an afternoon counselling workshop to a three-year educational programme. However, whatever the scale it is important to identify the tasks to be completed, the timescale for the completion, and those responsible for them.

Tasks for an evaluation usually follow three large-scale stages: planning and identifying questions; data collection; and analysis and reporting. The Steering Group is responsible overall for making sure these tasks are identified, allocated, and completed.

Gathering data to answer evaluation questions is the central activity of any programme evaluation. This needs to be project managed with clear objectives; a set time scale; completion date; and assigned responsibilities.

The Steering Group is responsible for project planning overall but with delegated responsibility to members. Given that the evaluation of the programme is the entire project, the Steering Group may wish to divide this large project into mini-projects; for example, gathering data for a particular outcome and each mini-project will also need to be managed. Obviously, evaluations vary in the number of staff available to complete projects which is largely dependent on resourcing and scheduling.

The main thing is to ensure that there are clear responsibilities for gathering the data, analysing the data, and creating the reports and recommendations to the Steering Group.

DOI: 10.4324/9781003312253-9

Case Study: Evaluation of a Community Partnership Service

INTRODUCTION

In contemporary programme evaluation, effective project management is no longer a peripheral concern—it is a central determinant of success. Evaluations are not mere academic exercises; they are time-sensitive, resource-bound, and multi-stakeholder projects. As such, they require structured planning, coherent oversight, and clear accountability. Without a sound management strategy, even the most methodologically sound evaluations can falter under the weight of unclear expectations, overlapping roles, or shifting service configurations.

This chapter explores practical strategies for managing evaluations using insights from a case study of a community partnership service. This case offers instructive lessons on structuring evaluation projects, managing evolving responsibilities, and maintaining momentum despite ambiguities in service design and delivery.

TREATING EVALUATIONS AS PROJECTS

Evaluations should be treated as formal projects in their own right. This means beginning with a scoping process that results in a documented evaluation plan. Such a plan should include clear objectives, timeframes, milestones, assigned responsibilities, and identified risks. The community partnership service evaluation was structured around the Trident Evaluation Model, which divided the evaluation into three key domains: outcomes, process, and stakeholder perspectives. Each domain functioned like a mini-project, with specific methods, deliverables, and assigned leads.

The segmentation of the evaluation into smaller, manageable components allowed the team to proceed methodically, even when one area encountered delays or access issues. For example, when data from administrative records proved incomplete, the team increased emphasis on interviews and case studies to maintain progress in the outcomes strand.

When breaking down a large evaluation, create a timeline for each mini-project, specifying dependencies (e.g., stakeholder interviews may depend on completion of a process map) and ensuring coordination between strands.

DEFINING SCOPE AND DELIVERABLES EARLY

Ambiguity about what exactly is being evaluated can derail progress. In this case, the absence of a detailed agreement for the service meant there was some confusion over what constituted formal service activity, who was responsible for recording it, and what quality standards were being applied. This vagueness created difficulties in both process and outcomes assessment.

To navigate this, the evaluators worked collaboratively with stakeholders to co-produce a set of evaluation objectives, drawing from policy documents, service descriptions, and practitioner insights. These objectives helped anchor the evaluation when formal documentation fell short.

Always supplement documentation review with stakeholder workshops or interviews early in the evaluation to define scope. Use this dialogue to fill gaps in formal records and secure buy-in.

ASSIGNING RESPONSIBILITIES ACROSS TEAMS

A central component of successful evaluation project management is clarity of roles. This evaluation featured a diverse set of actors: full-time and part-time workers, designated staff, programme managers, and external evaluators. The relationships between these actors were not straightforward, given that some were seconded from other agencies and operated under overlapping lines of accountability.

The evaluation team responded to this complexity by mapping out a responsibility matrix that specified who was responsible for delivering or supporting each aspect of the evaluation. This clarified, for example, who would coordinate interviews, who would ensure access to service documentation, and who would provide interim supervision for frontline staff contributing to the evaluation.

Develop a visual responsibility matrix early in the project. This helps ensure accountability and prevents duplicated effort or overlooked tasks.

INTEGRATING EVALUATION WITH SERVICE DELIVERY CONSTRAINTS

Many evaluations take place in live service environments with limited capacity for disruption. In the case study, the service under review was delivered flexibly via home visits, drop-in clinics, and informal conversations. This delivery model served vulnerable populations and prioritised accessibility. However, its informal nature created challenges for evaluators attempting to track client pathways, verify outcomes, or obtain systematic data.

Rather than imposing artificial structures, the evaluation team sought to understand and document the real-world dynamics of the service. For instance, they conducted "milling around" observations in drop-in sessions and built rapport with staff to gain insight into how issues emerged and were managed informally. They also used qualitative interviews with participants to fill the gaps left by inconsistent data recording practices.

Evaluate on the programme's own terms. Don't insist on data systems or documentation practices that clash with how the programme is delivered. Instead, triangulate evidence and use qualitative methods to uncover important findings that the numbers may overlook.

MANAGING RISKS AND CONTINGENCIES

Project management is ultimately about anticipating and adapting to uncertainty. In this evaluation, several risks materialised: staffing changes, service pauses, and ongoing tensions over the boundaries of certain roles. Rather than viewing these as disruptions, the evaluation team incorporated them into the narrative of the evaluation, documenting their implications for continuity, trust, and service outcomes.

A formal risk register was maintained throughout the project, with mitigation strategies that included shifting emphasis towards user perspectives when administrative data was unavailable and adapting the final reporting timeline when the programme status changed.

Do maintain a live issues log and risk register. Assign each risk an owner, track updates, and document what mitigation actions were taken. This not only helps manage the evaluation—it also enhances transparency and credibility.

THE IMPORTANCE OF COMMUNICATION AND RELATIONSHIP MANAGEMENT

Evaluation often involves navigating organisational boundaries. In the case study, the programme was delivered by workers seconded from one organisation into the premises and programs of another organization. These arrangements led to misalignments in expectations, particularly around supervision, data responsibilities, and day-to-day liaison.

The evaluation team managed this complexity by building strong relationships with key personnel in both organisations. Regular update meetings, informal check-ins, and feedback loops helped maintain access to information and mitigate tensions. For example, when evaluators needed clarification on client outcome tracking, they held parallel meetings with frontline workers and service managers to surface concerns that may not have emerged in a single joint session.

When working across agencies, invest time in stakeholder management. Build relationships at multiple levels of each organisation to ensure access to both operational detail and strategic direction.

REPORTING AS A PROCESS NOT A PRODUCT

One of the most effective project management strategies employed in the case study was treating reporting as a phased, integrated process rather than a final-stage task. Interim briefings were shared with programme staff and frontline workers to validate findings, test interpretations, and spark discussions about service improvement.

For example, early analysis of the lack of systematic data recording prompted discussions about what kinds of evidence were most helpful to staff. This in turn led to the development of simplified recording templates, co-produced with workers, which aimed to balance rigour with feasibility.

Use reporting as an engagement tool. Share early findings, ask for feedback, and demonstrate that the evaluation is a reflective and responsive process—not just a flat one-dimensional audit exercise.

LESSONS LEARNED FROM THE CASE

This evaluation illustrated the centrality of project management in achieving useful, credible results. Among the most salient lessons were:

- **Evaluations need structure but also flexibility.** Timelines and outputs should be defined early but evaluators must adapt as conditions change.
- **Relationship building is a genuine goal.** Managing interpersonal dynamics, especially in multi-agency contexts, is as crucial as data analysis.

- **Qualitative methods can fill systemic data gaps.** In settings with minimal formal tracking, client interviews, and narrative case studies can provide powerful evidence.
- **Evaluation should support learning not just judgement.** By integrating feedback into the process, evaluators help services improve in real time.

PRACTICAL RECOMMENDATIONS FOR EVALUATION PROJECT MANAGERS

1. **Co-produce the evaluation plan.** Work with stakeholders to define the purpose, boundaries, and outputs of the evaluation. Co-ownership reduces resistance and clarifies expectations.
2. **Use phased planning.** Break the evaluation into discrete components (e.g., design, data collection, analysis, reporting) with timelines, leads, and deliverables for each.
3. **Formalise responsibilities.** Whether through memoranda of understanding or internal tracking documents, clarify who is responsible for each evaluation task.
4. **Build in feedback loops.** Use early findings and interim reports to steer both the evaluation and the programme. Make learning part of the process.
5. **Anticipate and adapt to challenges.** Use a risk register, check-ins, and regular reflection to stay responsive to evolving service conditions.

CONCLUSION

Project management is not ancillary to programme evaluation—it is fundamental. When evaluators take the time to plan, assign responsibilities, monitor risks, and communicate effectively, they increase both the rigour and utility of their work. As this case illustrates, evaluations are most successful when they are planned and delivered with the same attention to detail, coordination, and reflection as any other professional project.

In a world of constrained budgets, time pressures, and complex partnerships, good project management practices are not just helpful—they are essential to generating useful, timely, and credible evaluation findings that inform future policy and practice.

CHAPTER 10

Determining outcomes with a case study of the evaluation of midwifery in community health

UNDERSTANDING OUTCOMES IN PROGRAMME EVALUATION

A fundamental question in programme evaluation is: *"Did it work?"* This seemingly simple question contains two distinct inquiries:

1. *Was the programme delivered as intended?* (Process)
2. *Did the programme lead to the desired changes in recipients*? (Outcomes)

While process focuses on how the programme was implemented, *outcomes* address whether it achieved its intended effects on participants.

DEFINING AND IDENTIFYING OUTCOMES

Programme providers often confuse delivery objectives with outcome objectives. However, outcomes should describe the *intended impact* on participants—changes in their behaviour, understanding, or attitudes—as a result of the programme.

A clear articulation of outcomes is typically required during programme planning especially when seeking funding or approval. These stated goals serve as a starting point for evaluation.

In preliminary evaluation stages providers are often asked:

"What outcomes should the programme be judged by?"

Answering this helps define success in terms of observable or measurable change.

EVIDENCE OF OUTCOMES

Once outcomes are defined, the next question is:

"What evidence will demonstrate that these outcomes have been achieved?"

DOI: 10.4324/9781003312253-10

This involves identifying appropriate indicators and deciding on methods to measure them. These methods—drawn from the social and behavioural sciences—may include surveys, interviews, behavioural observations, or other tools capable of capturing changes in beliefs, attitudes, or actions.

FEASIBILITY AND AGREEMENT

The *Steering Group* overseeing the evaluation must:

- Confirm that the selected outcomes accurately reflect the programme's aims.
- Ensure that generating valid, reliable evidence for these outcomes is feasible.

Outcomes must not only be meaningful but also measurable.

EXAMPLES IN PRACTICE

Each of the Trident model case studies illustrate how outcomes were specified and assessed in real-world evaluations, providing concrete examples of how to approach this key aspect of programme evaluation.

Case Study: Using the Trident Model on a Midwifery-Based Intervention in Community Health

INTRODUCTION

In the field of programme evaluation, assessing outcomes is crucial to determining the effectiveness and broader impact of an initiative. This chapter and case study explore the principles and practical application of outcomes evaluation, drawing on a detailed case study involving a midwifery intervention within a community-based maternal and infant health programme. While the example provided is anonymised, the findings are widely applicable across healthcare and social development contexts.

Using the Trident Evaluation Model—focusing on outcomes, processes, and multiple stakeholder perspectives—we delve into how to define, measure, and interpret outcomes in a rigorous and meaningful way. The evaluation examined here focused specifically on improving rates of breastfeeding, reducing maternal smoking, and promoting public health within a socioeconomically deprived community. It serves as a model of how outcomes can be approached in complex, multi-agency programs with evolving objectives.

DEFINING OUTCOMES IN EVALUATION

Outcomes represent the intended results or impacts of a programme. They differ from outputs, which are the immediate products of programme activities, and from processes, which refer to the methods and means by which a programme operates. Outcomes are typically defined in advance, either by funders, programme designers, or community stakeholders, and they should be framed in a way that allows for measurable progress over time.

In the context of the case study, the primary outcomes of interest were:

- Increased breastfeeding rates at birth, six weeks, and four months.
- Reduced rates of smoking in pregnancy.
- Higher rates of early contact with new and expectant mothers.
- Reduced incidence of low birthweight babies.

These outcomes aligned with national health objectives, as well as, local health inequalities strategies. Importantly, they were rooted in public health goals targeting early-life interventions, which research consistently identifies as critical for long-term well-being.

ESTABLISHING BASELINES AND TARGETS

A robust evaluation requires a clear baseline—a snapshot of relevant indicators before the intervention begins. Baseline data enables evaluators to compare before-and-after scenarios and to judge whether any observed changes are likely attributable to the programme.

In the example case study, baseline breastfeeding rates in the community were notably low, with only 7.6% of mothers breastfeeding at birth and even fewer at later stages. Similarly, 88% of pregnant women were smoking at the start of the programme. These figures provided a stark contrast against which the midwifery intervention could be measured.

Targets were then established: a 10% reduction in smoking during pregnancy and increased breastfeeding rates at all milestones. Setting targets not only helped in evaluation but also motivated programme staff by providing concrete goals.

USING QUANTITATIVE AND QUALITATIVE MEASURES

Outcomes evaluations benefit from a mix of quantitative and qualitative data. Quantitative data offers measurable, comparable figures—such as percentage changes or absolute numbers. Qualitative data adds depth, helping to explain why changes occurred or why certain targets were missed.

QUANTITATIVE DATA COLLECTED:

- Breastfeeding initiation and continuation rates.
- Smoking cessation rates at confirmation of pregnancy, six months, and nine months.
- Percentage of first-time mothers contacted during pregnancy.
- Rates of low birthweight births.
- Number of home and antenatal clinic visits conducted.

QUALITATIVE DATA COLLECTED:

- Interviews with midwives and programme staff.
- Focus groups with local health teams.
- Questionnaires distributed to programme participants (families).

This mixed-methods approach provided both the evidence of impact and insights into the mechanisms driving change.

MEASURING PROGRESS AND IMPACT

Breastfeeding outcomes

Breastfeeding rates were a core focus of the evaluation. The programme successfully increased rates at all stages. For example, the percentage of mothers breastfeeding at birth rose from 7.6% to over 30% by the end of the observation period. Continued breastfeeding at six weeks and four months also showed positive trends, though data was less complete.

Much of this progress can be attributed to the midwife's ability to deliver tailored, one-on-one support in the home, run educational antenatal groups, and initiate community-based campaigns, including a training programme for local peer support counsellors.

Smoking in pregnancy

Smoking cessation results were more mixed. While there was a notable drop in the percentage of women smoking during pregnancy—from 88% to 47%—longer-term cessation at six and nine months remained minimal. This suggests that while initial cessation messages were reaching women, maintaining abstinence was more challenging. It points to the importance of longer-term support mechanisms and perhaps the need for integrated behaviour-change models in future programme design.

Early engagement and low birth weight

Another successful outcome was the rate of early engagement with new mothers. From a baseline of 0%, the programme reached 100% of mothers within two months of birth during the evaluation period, largely due to the proactive efforts of the designated midwife.

The incidence of low birthweight babies also improved, falling from 9.1% to 1%. However, sample sizes were small, and while the improvement is promising, it should be interpreted with caution. Continued monitoring would be necessary to determine if this was part of a long-term trend.

INTERPRETING OUTCOMES WITHIN CONTEXT

While measurable outcomes provide important evidence of programme success, they must be interpreted within the broader social and organisational context.

In this case, several factors influenced outcomes:

- *Community Deprivation:* Health behaviours like smoking and breastfeeding are heavily influenced by social norms, cultural beliefs, and socioeconomic conditions. The midwife's community-based, relational approach helped overcome some of these barriers by building trust and continuity.

- *Service Integration:* The midwife worked alongside, but not always in coordination with, existing maternity services. This occasionally led to confusion for families and duplication of effort. Better service integration might have increased impact even further.
- *Evolving Role:* The midwife's responsibilities expanded during the programme, incorporating public health education in schools, supporting antenatal classes, and even engaging in governance activities. This evolution allowed for greater community impact but also raised questions about role clarity and sustainability.

ADDRESSING LIMITATIONS

Every evaluation must acknowledge its limitations. In this example, the following issues emerged:

- *Attribution Challenges:* Some outcomes, particularly increases in breastfeeding, may have also been influenced by hospital-based campaigns or broader national initiatives. Isolating the impact of the midwife's intervention is difficult in such a context.
- *Sample Size and Response Rate:* The family survey had a low response rate (14%), which limits the generalisability of findings. Nevertheless, responses were overwhelmingly positive, providing anecdotal validation of the intervention's effectiveness.
- *Data Management:* While data collection was robust, much of it was paper-based and lacked central integration. This made it harder to track trends systematically or to cross-verify data from different sources. Modern evaluations benefit greatly from digital monitoring systems.

LINKING OUTCOMES TO BROADER EVALUATION ELEMENTS

Using the Trident model, outcomes do not exist in isolation. They must be seen in relation to programme processes and stakeholder perspectives.

- *Processes:* The successful outcomes described were often underpinned by innovative practices—home visits, drop-in clinics, antenatal education, and peer support. Evaluators must track not just whether outcomes were achieved, but how.
- *Stakeholder Perspectives:* Interviews and focus groups revealed that the midwife's approach was deeply valued by families and fellow professionals, even where formal targets were not always met. This contextual understanding is vital for accurate interpretation of outcome data.

LESSONS FOR FUTURE EVALUATIONS

Based on the case study, several key lessons emerge for those planning and conducting evaluations:

1. *Define Outcomes Clearly and Early:* Ensure all stakeholders agree on what success looks like and how it will be measured.
2. *Use Mixed Methods:* Combine hard data with qualitative feedback to understand both outcomes and their drivers.
3. *Monitor Continuously:* Avoid one-off evaluations in favour of iterative data collection that can inform practice throughout the programme lifecycle.
4. *Involve Stakeholders:* Their insights can highlight overlooked impacts or contextual challenges not captured in standard metrics.
5. *Plan for Integration:* Programs that sit alongside existing services must carefully navigate roles and responsibilities to avoid duplication or confusion.
6. *Address Sustainability:* Roles that evolve beyond their initial remit, as in this case, should be supported by flexible governance and potential succession planning.

CONCLUSION

Outcomes-based evaluation offers a rigorous yet adaptable way to assess programme success, provided it is grounded in local realities and enriched with stakeholder insights. The case study of the community midwifery initiative highlights how targeted, relational interventions can shift entrenched public health behaviours, even in deprived settings.

By embedding outcomes evaluation within a broader framework—one that accounts for processes and stakeholder voices—evaluators and programme designers can more accurately assess what works, for whom, and under what conditions. The lessons derived from this example extend far beyond healthcare, offering valuable guidance for any outcome-focused intervention seeking to make meaningful and measurable change.

CHAPTER 11

Process

Capturing, recording, and analysing process in programme evaluation with a case study of a mental healthcare collaborative

Process refers to the actions of the provider in delivering the programme. It includes the organisation of individuals (primarily) and materials and activities.

The description of this process should be sufficiently detailed to allow the programme to be repeated and also to allow the identification of variables which are associated with the outcomes.

Starting points for the process would be the response to the preliminary questionnaire and documented descriptions for the implementation of the process, particularly if it represented a significant change in previous practice.

These documented descriptions must meet the standard of allowing the process to be replicated. They should allow preliminary hypotheses to be formulated linking the process with specified outcomes.

While documented descriptions make a good starting point the programme evaluation should gather its own data on process or, at the very least, verify the documentary evidence. Further investigations can reveal more details and could well suggest hypotheses regarding relationships with outcomes or stakeholder perspectives that would otherwise have gone unnoticed.

Process can be researched in various ways. Observation of process is one method but is beset with many logistical and ethical problems. Another approach involves the providers themselves in reflection and analysis and can be very productive. This method been used to construct a valid description or ethnography of process and has been termed reconstituted ethnography. Recollections and reflections are recorded and organised by the researchers then verified by the participants.

DOI: 10.4324/9781003312253-11

Ultimately, evaluating process is not only about documenting what was done but about understanding how and why those actions contributed to—or hindered—the programme's intended outcomes. A robust process analysis enhances the credibility, transferability, and depth of a programme evaluation.

Case Study: An Evaluation of a Mental Healthcare Collaborative

Effective programme evaluation requires more than evidence of outcomes. To fully understand how and why a programme works—or fails to—it is essential to evaluate its processes. This chapter provides a practical, research-informed guide to capturing, recording, and analysing the processes of a programme and systematically linking them to outcomes. Using a case study evaluation of a Mental Healthcare Collaborative (MHC), we explore methods for collecting and interpreting process data and integrating this with outcome findings to support programme learning, refinement, and replication.

Understanding process is not simply about identifying activities; it involves tracing the pathways by which inputs become outputs and outcomes. These pathways include human interactions, decision-making frameworks, inter-organisational dynamics, and changes in user experience. Process evaluation enables evaluators to ask and answer critical questions: how is the programme delivered in practice? Are processes coherent, consistent, and responsive? What unintended effects are produced along the way? And ultimately, how do these processes contribute to—or hinder—intended outcomes?

The MHC case study offers a valuable illustration of how such questions can be approached systematically in complex, multi-agency service settings.

DEFINING AND SPECIFYING PROCESS IN COMPLEX PROGRAMS

Process evaluation begins with specification. Evaluators must first understand the operational logic of the programme: its design, delivery mechanisms, organisational structures, and intended service pathways. In the MHC evaluation, this involved modelling the programme's referral, assessment, intervention, and discharge stages, as well as, its training and stakeholder engagement activities. These were mapped against a client journey, with specific milestones and mechanisms identified at each stage.

A common challenge in complex programmes is vague or inconsistent process documentation. MHC initially lacked formalised procedures in areas such as consultation or inter-agency coordination, which made replication difficult. Evaluation fieldwork helped clarify these gaps, prompting the development of shared protocols and assessment tools. Early specification of processes not only supports evaluation but helps teams reflect on and codify their own practice.

To be useful, process specifications must also be sufficiently detailed to enable replication. For example, in the MHC model, structured referral meetings and multidisciplinary decision-making processes were described in terms of their membership, timing, and rules of decisions. Such detail supports fidelity analysis: the extent to which implementation aligns with design.

CAPTURING PROCESS: DATA SOURCES AND INSTRUMENTS

Capturing process data requires a multi-method approach. The MHC evaluation used interviews, focus groups, document review, observation, and administrative data to record process flows. Each method played a distinct role:

- **Semi-structured interviews** were conducted with staff at all levels to understand roles, inter-professional relationships, and perceived strengths and weaknesses of delivery processes.
- **Focus groups** with frontline workers explored shared norms and informal practices that shaped client engagement.
- **Document analysis** of referral forms, assessment tools, supervision records, and training logs provided a basis for mapping structured processes.
- **Observations** of referral and review meetings helped triangulate reported practices with actual behaviours.
- **Monthly "staff return forms"** offered quantitative data on consultation, supervision, training, and client contact volumes.

The strength of this approach lies in its triangulation: no single data source is adequate, but taken together they offer a rich, composite picture. For instance, interviews revealed a desire for greater consistency in assessment, while document analysis showed that standardised tools were underused. The evaluation team was then able to recommend tighter alignment between stated protocols and everyday practice.

To maximise credibility, evaluators must be transparent about data limitations. In the MHC case, under-completion of return forms limited the evaluators' ability to measure progress towards certain outcome indicators. These data quality issues became part of the process findings themselves, prompting discussions about the need for improved data culture and infrastructure.

ANALYSING PROCESS DATA: FROM DESCRIPTION TO INTERPRETATION

Capturing process is only the first step; analysis requires interpretation of how processes affect both users and outcomes. A key analytic tool in the MHC evaluation was the use of *process maps*, developed from documentary and interview data, to depict care pathways. These maps showed not only formal steps but also decision points, feedback loops, and bottlenecks. For instance, the referral process was depicted as a weekly triage system involving representatives from psychological care, probation services, housing, and multiple other agencies.

The process maps were then cross-referenced with client outcomes and stakeholder perceptions. One critical insight was the impact of consistent referral team membership on decision quality. Previously, inconsistent attendance had led to variability in decisions; after the introduction of a "core team" model, decisions became more predictable and aligned with programme objectives.

Another analytical strategy was the categorisation of *intervention types* and their relational characteristics. The MHC offered multiple forms of engagement—from therapeutic work grounded in psychoanalytic frameworks to social support activities like housing advocacy or skills training. By coding interviews and case notes, evaluators were able to distinguish between directive and non-directive approaches, and assess how each related to client retention, engagement, and satisfaction.

Quantitative analysis of process data was also valuable. Monthly figures on client contacts, cancellations, and training sessions provided a numeric basis for understanding activity levels and workload distribution. However, these numbers only became meaningful when interpreted in context. For example, a rise in cancelled appointments prompted analysis of external stressors affecting clients and suggested a need to build more flexibility into care plans.

LINKING PROCESS AND OUTCOMES: A SYSTEMATIC APPROACH

A central challenge in any evaluation is *linking what was done (process) to what was achieved (outcomes)*. In the MHC case, the evaluation adopted a "logic-informed" framework: outcomes were traced backward to the activities and decisions that contributed to them. This was not a strict causal model but an effort to establish plausible connections between process patterns and outcome trajectories.

For instance, MHC's emphasis on service user involvement—reflected in events, newsletters, and advisory roles—was linked to improved perceptions of empowerment and inclusion amongst clients. Similarly, the establishment of out-of-hours support pathways was related to reduced emergency service usage, although attribution remained cautious due to limited control data.

The evaluators also examined how *variation in process* led to differential outcomes. Clients whose assessment followed the newly structured X-week model showed higher rates of continuing engagement than those assessed under the older, more ad hoc system. These findings supported further investment in structured assessment protocols.

The use of *repeated measures*—e.g., client wellbeing scores at baseline(X), X+1, X+2, and X+3 weeks—allowed tracking of individual trajectories. Although outcome improvements could not be conclusively attributed to specific interventions, the data highlighted promising associations, such as the correlation between consistent contact with support workers and reduced cancellations.

Importantly, the evaluation did not assume that all processes should or could be standardised. Flexibility was often key to engagement, particularly for clients with complex needs. The analytic task was to identify which elements of flexibility supported outcomes and which introduced risk or inconsistency.

PROCESS LEARNING: REFINING PRACTICE THROUGH EVALUATION

One of the most important functions of process evaluation is organisational learning. By making delivery visible, evaluation creates opportunities for reflection and improvement. In the MHC case, the evaluation process itself prompted several adaptations:

- Referral procedures were clarified; with referrers receiving forms in advance to enhance information quality.
- Communication between therapists and care coordinators was improved via regular case review meetings.
- The network implemented a discharge panel to bring greater structure and accountability to transitions.

These changes were not merely administrative; they reflected a broader shift towards *intentional practice*. Staff began to articulate the "why" behind their actions, leading to more consistent and coherent service delivery.

At the system level, evaluation findings were fed into local commissioning discussions and were used to advocate for the continuation and expansion of MHC-like services. Process findings—particularly the emphasis on cross-agency collaboration—were cited in strategic planning documents as models of integrated care.

PRACTICAL GUIDANCE FOR EVALUATORS

Based on the MHC case, the following principles are recommended for evaluators seeking to capture and relate process to outcomes:

1. *Start with Specification*: Clarify intended processes early in the evaluation. If the programme lacks formal process documents assist and support teams to articulate their working models.
2. *Use Multiple Data Sources*: Combine interviews, observations, documents, and administrative data. No single method will suffice especially in a complex area and system.
3. *Triangulate Rigorously*: Compare what people say, what documents show, and what actually happens.
4. *Develop Process Maps*: Visual representations can clarify complex pathways and highlight critical junctures.
5. *Quantify Where Possible*: Use numeric data to track volume, frequency, and timing—but always interpret in context.
6. *Analyse Variation*: Identify when and why processes deviate and how this affects outcomes.
7. *Link Backward from Outcomes*: Trace what processes preceded success or failure, looking for patterns.
8. *Embed Learning*: Share interim findings with teams to support adaptation during the evaluation.
9. *Respect Complexity*: Avoid oversimplification. Processes in human services are often non-linear and mediated by relationships.
10. *Document Changes*: Track how the programme evolves over time, especially if prompted by the evaluation itself.

CONCLUSION

Process evaluation is not merely an adjunct to outcome analysis; it is a critical perspective for understanding how programmes function in practice. By capturing, recording, and analysing processes, evaluators illuminate the mechanisms that drive results, the conditions that support success, and the adaptations that will enable sustainability. The MHC case shows that such work requires commitment to detail, openness to complexity, and a belief that transparency in process is a foundation for meaningful change.

In summary, systematic attention to process allows programme teams not only to ask: "*Did it work?*" but to understand why, how, and for whom it worked—and to improve practice accordingly.

CHAPTER 12

Understanding and integrating multiple stakeholder perspectives in programme evaluation

A case study of a comprehensive cancer support network (CCSN)

The third prong of the of the Trident—multiple stakeholder perspectives—is complementary to the other two prongs in several ways.

First, it gives an opportunity to all those involved in the programme, either directly or indirectly, to express a view on the programme.

Second, the data methodologically tends to be more qualitative than the other prongs which are characterised by a more scientific approach with hard data which is quantitative whenever possible.

Third, it can give a perspective on the programme which is complementary or sometimes even contradictory to the other two prongs. For example, a medical programme may appear to be very effective through the accomplishment of measurable outcomes and through its professional style of delivery. But the views of the participants may be quite different. For instance, a mobility programme might increase the range of movement or measurable outcome but might make the patient feel that they have lost personal autonomy and self-determination.

Who then are the stakeholders? It is useful for the Steering Group to reflect on a 360° analysis of those involved in the programme. They will include, obviously, the participants and the providers, but also managers to whom the providers are responsible and representatives of participants or even community members from the programme setting.

As in the other prongs, a range of research methods are available to sample the views of stakeholders: interviews, focus groups, and questionnaires can be valuable. The emphasis is on capturing the subjective perceptions of participants which can be compared and contrasted with the data gathered more objectively regarding outcomes and processes.

DOI: 10.4324/9781003312253-12

Case study of the Evaluation: A Comprehensive Cancer Support Network (CCSN)

INTRODUCTION

Stakeholder perspectives are a critical component of an extensive programme evaluation. Their integration not only ensures inclusivity and transparency but also contributes significantly to the depth and validity of evaluation findings. This guide explores practical methods and principles for incorporating multiple stakeholder perspectives into the evaluation. Drawing on an anonymised case study involving a CCSN, this guide illustrates how stakeholder insights can be systematically collected, analysed, and used to enhance both service delivery and evaluation practice.

WHY STAKEHOLDER PERSPECTIVES MATTER

Stakeholders represent the numerous groups with a vested interest in the programme under evaluation. These include direct service participants, front-line practitioners, programme coordinators and managers, policymakers, and in some cases, associated organisations such as partner institutions or advocacy groups. Each brings unique insights shaped by their experiences, responsibilities, and expectations.

Incorporating multiple stakeholder perspectives:

- Provides a more complete understanding of how a programme operates in practice.
- Reveals discrepancies between intended and actual service delivery.
- Identifies areas of strength and opportunity from diverse viewpoints.
- Builds trust and engagement among stakeholders.
- Supports sustainability by involving those affected in shaping future iterations.

IDENTIFYING RELEVANT STAKEHOLDERS

The first step in collecting stakeholder perspectives is identifying the many stakeholders involved in the programme. This may seem straightforward, but in practice, evaluators must think expansively. In the case study, the following groups were identified:

- **Service users (patients)** who experienced the programme directly.
- **Care coordinators and nurses**, who implemented care plans and had ongoing contact with users.
- **Programme managers and lead clinicians**, responsible for strategy, oversight, and staff development.
- **Primary care teams**, including general practitioners involved in collaborative care.
- **Specialist clinical staff**, such as consultants or specialist nurses involved in education and case support.
- **Health system representatives**, who had a macro-level view of resource allocation and regional integration.

A mapping process—sometimes visual—is useful to organise stakeholder categories and levels of influence, helping evaluators ensure broad and thorough representation.

METHODS FOR GATHERING STAKEHOLDER DATA

To collect perspectives effectively, evaluators should apply a combination of qualitative and quantitative methods. The selected methods must be accessible, ethically sound, and tailored to each group's context and availability.

Interviews and focus groups

Semi-structured interviews and focus groups provide rich, qualitative insights. In the case study, interviews were conducted with district nurses, programme coordinators, and management staff. Focus groups were also held with front-line clinical teams.

Advantages:

- Allow exploration of experiences in depth.
- Facilitate clarification and follow-up on nuanced issues.
- Can reveal emotional and contextual dimensions often absent from surveys.

Challenges:

- Require time and skilled facilitators.
- May be constrained by participants' availability and openness.

Practical Tip: Use open-ended questions and prompts that allow for reflection on both operational and emotional aspects of service delivery. Ensure confidentiality and comfort for participants.

Patient surveys

Structured surveys distributed to service users provided a means to collect data from a wider pool. In this case, surveys were sent to a group of cancer patients enrolled in the CCSN. A nearly 50% response rate was achieved.

Advantages:

- Cost-effective method for capturing large sample views.
- Enable statistical analysis of trends and frequencies.
- Useful for standardising questions across settings.

Challenges:

- Limited depth; may miss context.
- Potential non-response bias, particularly among disengaged or dissatisfied participants.

Practical Tip: Include both closed and open-ended questions to balance standardisation with richness. Pilot test the instrument with a small group before full distribution.

Documentary analysis

Reviewing documents such as meeting minutes, care pathways, training records, and previous evaluations provides context and corroborates stakeholder claims. This was used to assess implementation fidelity in the case study.

Advantages:

- Non-intrusive and readily available.
- Complements, interviews, and surveys.

Challenges:

- May be incomplete or inconsistent.
- Risk of over-interpreting formal documentation.

Practical Tip: Triangulate documentary evidence with stakeholder accounts to identify convergences and discrepancies.

ANALYSING AND SYNTHESISING STAKEHOLDER DATA

Collecting stakeholder views is only the beginning. Evaluators must also make sense of the data in ways that reflect the complexity and diversity of perspectives.

THEMATIC ANALYSIS

Thematic analysis is especially well-suited to qualitative data. In the case study, recurring themes such as "reassurance and support," "coordination of care," and "communication challenges" were identified through repeated readings of interview transcripts and focus group notes.

Steps:

1. Transcribe all interviews/focus group sessions.
2. Read through for initial impressions.
3. Code significant statements.
4. Group codes into themes.
5. Validate themes with secondary reviewers or through respondent validation.

TRIANGULATION

Triangulation strengthens the credibility of findings by comparing results across data types (e.g., interviews, surveys, and documents) or stakeholder groups. For instance, patients in the case study overwhelmingly appreciated having a single point of contact, and this was echoed in interviews with staff.

Triangulation types:

- **Methodological** (e.g., survey + interview).
- **Data source** (e.g., patients vs. staff).
- **Theoretical** (applying different lenses to the data).

CONTRADICTIONS AND DIVERGENCE

Not all stakeholder perspectives align. Patients in the evaluation highlighted issues with messaging systems and inconsistent follow-up, while some staff believed systems were functioning adequately. Rather than obscuring these divergences, evaluators should highlight them, as they indicate areas for deeper inquiry and possible programme improvement.

Case Study Insights: Themes from Multiple Stakeholder Perspectives

The following themes emerged from the stakeholder data in the case study. These illustrate how perspectives can shape and enhance evaluation insights.

ENHANCED PATIENT EXPERIENCE

Service users reported high levels of satisfaction, particularly valuing the single point of contact and the continuity of care provided. Over 70% of patients described contact arrangements as excellent or very good, and qualitative comments underscored the reassurance of having someone available during a period of uncertainty.

PROFESSIONAL CONFIDENCE AND CHALLENGES

Staff viewed the integration model positively, particularly the expanded role of district nurses and their access to targeted training. However, challenges included difficulty accessing training due to workload and scheduling limitations.

This suggests that while stakeholder support was high, practical constraints still required attention.

SYSTEM COORDINATION

Stakeholders generally agreed that the programme improved the coordination of services. Patients felt that their CCSN nurse helped them get the care they needed from multiple professionals. However, some raised concerns about gaps in communication or delays in responses to queries.

PROGRAMME SCALABILITY AND FUTURE USE

Across all professional groups, there was support for adapting the model to other chronic conditions. The shared belief was that the framework—particularly the care coordination and holistic assessment—could be extended to patients with long-term conditions like heart failure or diabetes.

ETHICAL CONSIDERATIONS IN ENGAGING STAKEHOLDERS

Engaging stakeholders in programme evaluations must be handled ethically. Participants must be informed about the purpose of the evaluation, consent must be obtained, and confidentiality should be maintained. In the case study, staff consented to recorded interviews, and patient surveys were anonymous and approved through governance procedures.

Best practices:

- Gain informed consent for participation and data use.
- Ensure participants can withdraw at any time.
- Provide participants with summaries of findings if appropriate.

INCORPORATING STAKEHOLDER FEEDBACK INTO RECOMMENDATIONS

Evaluation is not just about gathering data—it's about using it. Stakeholder input should be reflected in final reports, particularly when forming recommendations.

From the case study, areas for development included:

- Improving access to phone and messaging systems.
- Streamlining documentation processes to reduce burden on nurses.
- Expanding access to training.
- Ensuring better communication across clinical teams.

By explicitly linking these recommendations to stakeholder views, evaluators demonstrate responsiveness and build credibility.

CONCLUSION: EMBEDDING STAKEHOLDER ENGAGEMENT IN EVALUATION PRACTICE

Stakeholder engagement is not an optional add-on to evaluation—it is a foundational element. By systematically including diverse perspectives, evaluators can illuminate complex dynamics, increase the relevance of findings, and produce actionable recommendations. The anonymised case study discussed in this guide illustrates both the opportunities and challenges in collecting and analysing stakeholder perspectives. Through thoughtful planning, ethical practice, and a commitment to inclusivity, evaluators can ensure that the voices of all those affected by a programme are heard—and that their insights drive meaningful improvements.

KEY TAKEAWAYS

- Identify a wide range of stakeholders early in the evaluation process.
- Use mixed methods (surveys, interviews, documents) to gather comprehensive data.
- Analyse data thematically and triangulate across sources to enhance credibility.
- Highlight both convergences and contradictions in perspectives.
- Use stakeholder feedback to inform practical and policy-relevant recommendations.
- Maintain ethical standards throughout the engagement process.

CHAPTER 13

Reporting in programme evaluation

With a case study of structuring, communicating, and using findings from a nurse education initiative

Reporting is a critical thread running through every phase of a programme evaluation. Far from being a one-off activity at the end, reporting should be an iterative and strategic process that both informs and shapes the evaluation as it unfolds. When thoughtfully planned and executed, reporting not only communicates findings but also actively supports decision-making, stakeholder engagement, and continuous quality improvement.

At key milestones, interim reports should provide timely feedback to the Steering Group or oversight body. These formative reports enable real-time reflection, adjustment, and shared learning—ensuring that emerging insights are not lost but integrated into practice. Reports tied to specific sub-projects or workstreams also help maintain momentum and accountability across complex or multi-strand evaluations.

The final, or summative, report is more than a retrospective summary—it serves as a bridge to action. It should consolidate data in response to the agreed evaluation questions, draw clear conclusions, and present actionable recommendations. Ideally, it should hold no surprises for stakeholders who have remained engaged throughout the process. This underscores the importance of continuous reporting and collaborative reflection.

All reports—interim and summative—should include not only the data and analysis, but also proposals for action, naming responsible parties and setting timescales. Reporting is not an end but a means to improvement. Whether the report feeds internal strategy, supports service redesign, or underpins academic or professional publications, it must be clear, credible, and accessible to its intended audiences. Considerations of confidentiality and appropriate circulation must also be addressed by the Steering Group and Programme Evaluators.

Ultimately, effective reporting is foundational to a successful programme evaluation. It ensures transparency, builds trust, and facilitates real-world impact.

DOI: 10.4324/9781003312253-13

Case Study: Evaluating the Communication and Reporting of the Findings of a Nurse Education Initiative

INTRODUCTION

Reporting is a foundational element of programme evaluation. It serves as the key mechanism by which data is transformed into actionable knowledge. While the collection and analysis of information are essential, it is through reporting that the programme evaluation becomes a useful instrument for informing decisions, guiding improvements, and shaping policy. Reporting should not be relegated to a final administrative task. Rather, it must be embedded throughout the evaluation cycle, with attention given to interim and summative stages alike. In doing so, programme evaluators ensure that stakeholders remain informed, engaged, and able to benefit from the evaluation process.

This chapter outlines how to effectively design and deliver programme evaluation reports. Drawing on practical experience, it incorporates lessons learned from the evaluation of a Nurse Education Initiative. This case study illustrates how purposeful reporting supported clarity, accountability, and ultimately the improvement of both education practice and policy.

THE ROLE OF REPORTING IN EVALUATION

The purpose and importance of reporting

Reporting serves several crucial functions. First, it ensures transparency in the evaluation process by clearly communicating what was done, how it was done, and what was found. Second, it provides a mechanism for accountability, enabling funders, managers, and other stakeholders to verify whether objectives were achieved. Third, reporting fosters learning and knowledge translation. By conveying findings in a structured and accessible format, evaluators help stakeholders apply insights to real-world contexts.

Well-constructed reports support reflective practice, allowing organisations to refine their interventions based on evidence. They also act as reference points for future programming helping to document progress over time. Furthermore, clear and honest reporting builds trust in the evaluation process itself and can open pathways to systemic or policy change.

Timing and phases of reporting

Reporting should occur at distinct stages during the evaluation process. Initial reports typically establish the evaluation's scope, goals, and methodology. These foundational documents set expectations and confirm alignment among programme evaluators and stakeholders.

Interim reports serve a formative function, providing updates on early findings and emerging trends. They can prompt timely adjustments to the programme or to the evaluation design itself. Regular reporting of this kind promotes responsiveness and collaboration particularly in complex or evolving programmes.

Final, or summative, reports consolidate all findings and deliver evidence-based conclusions. These reports often inform strategic decisions, justify continued funding, or highlight areas for further investment. In this case study, although the final report was a focal point, the importance of earlier, formative communication could also be seen in the way the evaluation responded to stakeholder concerns during implementation.

STRUCTURING EVALUATION REPORTS

An effective programme evaluation report should be logical, comprehensive, and tailored to its intended audience. The following components are recommended as best practice:

A. **Executive Summary**
   The executive summary is the most frequently read section of any report, particularly by senior leaders and decision-makers. It must succinctly present the purpose of the evaluation, the methods used, the major findings, and the key recommendations. In the case study, the executive summary effectively highlighted how the new curriculum improved clinical readiness among students and enhanced the integration between academic instruction and professional practice.

B. **Introduction and Background**
   The introduction should clearly set the scene by outlining the context in which the evaluation was conducted. This includes a description of the programme or initiative under review, its intended outcomes, and the motivations for undertaking the evaluation. In the case study, the initiative stemmed from national reforms intended to improve nurse education with particular focus on bridging the gap between theoretical instruction and clinical competence. The background section also offers space to acknowledge relevant policy developments, institutional goals, or historical concerns that shaped the programme.

C. **Evaluation Questions and the Trident Model**
   A central organising feature of any evaluation report is the articulation of evaluation questions. These questions often follow a structured model such as the Trident framework, which addresses outcomes, processes, and multiple stakeholder perspectives. In the case study evaluation, key questions included whether the new curriculum was perceived to be more effective than its predecessor, how well it integrated theoretical and practical elements, and what academic staff considered to be its most significant achievements and challenges. Clearly stated questions help readers understand the report's scope and purpose while also guiding the interpretation of results.

D. **Methods and Design**

The credibility of an evaluation depends greatly on the transparency and rigour of its methods. This section should provide a thorough account of the evaluation design, data sources, sampling strategies, and analytic techniques. In the case study, the evaluation employed a mixed-methods survey distributed to all nursing and midwifery academic staff and students. The questionnaires included both closed-ended items for statistical analysis and open-ended questions that captured qualitative insights. With a notably high response rate, the data collected offered both breadth and depth; thereby, enhancing the reliability of the findings.

E. **Presentation of Results**

The results section should be presented in a structured manner, typically aligned with the evaluation questions. Quantitative findings can be summarised through tables, charts, and narrative explanations. Qualitative data should be synthesised into themes or categories with illustrative anonymised quotes as appropriate.

In the case study evaluation, the results revealed that staff overwhelmingly viewed the new curriculum as a significant improvement over the previous model. Key positive findings included better preparation of students for clinical practice and stronger alignment between theory and practice. However, areas of concern also emerged, including dissatisfaction with modularisation, concerns about student workload, and perceptions of limited resources and placements. The clarity and organisation of these results allowed stakeholders to grasp the complexity of the programme's implementation and impact.

F. **Discussion and Interpretation**

Beyond presenting data, the discussion section should interpret the findings in light of the original evaluation questions and the broader context. This involves considering the implications of the results, identifying patterns or inconsistencies, and exploring potential reasons behind the findings.

In the case study evaluation, the discussion acknowledged the curriculum's positive impact on student preparedness and professional competence while recognising that excessive assessment and fragmented module structures hindered student experience. These interpretations were not merely descriptive but also provided explanatory insights that could inform curriculum revisions and broader institutional reforms.

G. **Evidence-Based Conclusions**

Conclusions must be rooted in the evidence presented. They should summarise what the evaluation has revealed and clarify what can be said with confidence. In this case, conclusions pointed to the initiative's success in meeting several key objectives, particularly in enhancing clinical learning and professional development. At the same time, the evaluation did not shy away from highlighting deficiencies in resource allocation, assessment design, and module integration.

Conclusions that are both candid and grounded in data increase the report's credibility and practical value.

H. **Recommendations**

Recommendations should be actionable, realistic, and directly linked to the evaluation's findings. Rather than simply listing areas for improvement, quality recommendations explain how identified issues might be addressed and by whom while also highlighting strengths that need to remain and receive continued support.

In the case study, recommendations included reviewing the module structure to improve coherence, reducing the overall assessment burden particularly in the early years, and expanding placement opportunities to meet student learning needs. These recommendations were informed by both staff and student feedback and statistical analysis ensuring that they addressed genuine and documented concerns.

COMMUNICATING WITH DIFFERENT AUDIENCES

Evaluation reports must be tailored to suit different stakeholders. While a full technical report is essential for internal and archival purposes, summary briefs, presentations, and policy memos may be more effective for certain audiences.

Technical reports are usually comprehensive and detailed, including full descriptions of methods, data tables, and appendices. These are suited to academic or research-oriented audiences.

Policy briefs, on the other hand, distil key findings and recommendations into two or three pages and are designed to influence decision-making. Presentations and workshops provide opportunities for dialogue and immediate feedback, helping stakeholders engage with findings in a more dynamic manner.

In this case, the primary audience included academic staff and faculty administrators, but the report also had implications for national education policymakers. Multiple formats have supported more widespread dissemination and utility of the programme evaluation's insights.

FORMATIVE AND SUMMATIVE REPORTING

Effective evaluations use both formative and summative reporting to ensure relevance throughout the evaluation cycle.

Formative reports, often delivered during the early or middle stages, can alert programme managers to emerging trends or unanticipated issues. While not formal documents, they serve a critical role in helping stakeholders make timely adjustments.

Although this evaluation focused on summative reporting, one could infer the value that ongoing feedback and informal discussions might have had in addressing concerns such as student workload or module alignment.

Summative reports, by contrast, provide a complete account of the evaluation. They consolidate findings, offer final conclusions, and serve as enduring records for future reference. In this case, the final report functioned as both an evaluative document and a planning tool, offering structured insights that could inform future curriculum development.

SUPPORTING PRACTICE IMPROVEMENT THROUGH REPORTING

One of the principal goals of reporting is to support improvement in practice. This involves more than identifying problems; it means framing findings in ways that facilitate reflection, learning, and change.

In the case study report, programme evaluators were careful to highlight successful innovations—such as the introduction of new modes of assessment and enhanced clinical skills development—even as they pointed out areas needing revision. This balanced approach helped staff appreciate the strengths of the initiative while remaining open to its limitations. Such framing encourages constructive responses and makes it more likely that recommendations will be adopted and success will be maintained.

REPORTING FOR POLICY INFLUENCE

When programmes operate within policy-sensitive environments, evaluation reports can be important tools for shaping or reinforcing policy direction. To maximise policy relevance reports should link findings to policy objectives, use appropriate terminology, and clearly demonstrate how the programme contributes to broader system-level goals.

In this case, the programme was introduced in response to national reforms in health education. The programme evaluation report; therefore, had the potential to influence future decisions at both institutional and national levels. By aligning its conclusions with the original aims of the reform, the evaluation lent credibility to the initiative and provided useful feedback to policymakers.

STYLE, LANGUAGE, AND PRESENTATION

The quality of writing and presentation plays a vital role in how evaluation findings are received. Reports should be written in clear, accessible language, avoiding technical jargon unless required by the audience. Visual aids such as charts and graphs can enhance understanding but should always be accompanied by explanatory text.

Well-organised sections, clear headings, and summary boxes at the end of major parts can guide readers and reinforce key messages. In this evaluation, the combination of quantitative graphs and qualitative summaries contributed to an engaging and informative report.

ETHICAL CONSIDERATIONS

Reporting must adhere to ethical standards. This includes maintaining participant confidentiality, accurately representing findings, and acknowledging limitations. Programme evaluators must also be transparent about their roles, funding sources, and any potential conflicts of interest.

In the case study, ethical integrity was maintained by anonymising responses, presenting aggregate data, and including both strengths and criticisms of the programme. Such practices build trust and support the legitimacy of the evaluation process.

CONCLUSION

Reporting is the capstone of any evaluation but it is also integral to every stage of the evaluation process. Thoughtful, structured, and ethical reporting not only documents what has been learned but enables that knowledge to be applied. The case study illustrates how rigorous reporting can translate complex findings into meaningful insights for practitioners, educators, and policymakers alike.

When preparing your own programme evaluation reports, consider not only what you have learned but also how best to communicate them. Effective reporting ensures that evaluations do not remain static documents but become catalysts for learning and growth.

CHAPTER 14

Impact on policy and practice

Case Study: Evaluation of an international social work student placement

In Chapter 1, we explored the benefits of programme evaluation for both providers and participants. Here, we turn our attention inward, reflecting on what motivates evaluators—drawing from our own experience in the hope that our reflections resonate with readers. At its core, we see evaluation as inseparable from the pursuit of improvement, regardless of the scale or scope of the programme.

We hold a strong belief that the outcomes of evaluation can meaningfully influence both practice and policy. Evaluation is not merely an exercise in critique; it is a constructive process aimed at uncovering areas for development and identifying practical solutions and also highlighting success for continuation and replication. While addressing evaluation questions may expose shortcomings, it is the evaluator's responsibility to move beyond identification and propose actionable recommendations—clearly outlining what should be done, by whom, and within what timeframe.

These recommendations are not made in isolation. They should emerge from a collaborative process, agreed upon by the evaluation's Steering Group, incorporating insights from service providers alongside the independent perspective of external evaluators. This ensures that recommendations are not only well-informed but also practically grounded and acceptable to stakeholders.

Formative evaluations, conducted during programme delivery, can include interim recommendations to enhance implementation. Final reports, in turn, should offer guidance not only on improving practice but also on shaping the broader policies within which these practices operate. The Steering Group plays a key role in this process—responsible for specifying responsibilities and timescales for implementing recommendations, and ideally, reconvening after a set period to review progress.

Another motivating factor in programme evaluation is the opportunity that programme evaluation provides to apply and refine research methods developed in the social and behavioural sciences. In this way, evaluation breathes life into theoretical

DOI: 10.4324/9781003312253-14

knowledge, offering rich material for research training, dissertations, and academic inquiry.

Ultimately, we believe that a core motivation for conducting evaluations should be the desire to support and improve the services being delivered. We hope this book inspires programme providers to initiate evaluations of their own practice—not out of obligation but from a genuine commitment to enhancement.

Improving practice—and the policy context in which it is embedded—is, in our view, the primary motivation behind all programme evaluation. This motivation is closely tied to the fundamental nature of work in education, health, and social care, which aims to improve individual lives, communities, and the nature of society.

Case Study: The Evaluation of an International Social Work Student Placement

INTRODUCTION: WHY FOCUS ON POLICY AND PRACTICE?

Evaluating the impact of a programme on policy and practice is often the most difficult yet arguably the most important aspect of a comprehensive evaluation. While assessing outcomes and processes helps measure effectiveness and understand delivery, focusing on policy and practice moves beyond measurement into application. It addresses the question: "What now?" How do we use what we have learned to inform future decision-making, shape institutional practice, and refine professional standards?

This guide draws on the evaluation of an international social care placement initiative involving social policy and social work students from a European university placed in a community care setting in the United Kingdom and linked to a local university. Using this pilot evaluation, we explore practical ways evaluators can identify, trace, and support the real-world application of findings into both policy development and practice transformation.

SETTING THE SCENE: FROM EVALUATION TO ACTION

Effective evaluation does not end with reporting results. To ensure an evaluation influences policy and practice, evaluators must:

- Understand the political and institutional context.
- Identify key audiences for recommendations.
- Communicate findings accessibly.
- Build pathways for implementation and follow-up.

These principles were put into action in the international placement pilot, where a group of students undertook social care placements in community service departments. The evaluation explicitly aimed to consider not only the outcomes of the placements, but also how learnings could inform future transnational partnerships, improve student support mechanisms, and develop local capacity to work with international professionals.

FRAMING RECOMMENDATIONS FOR IMPACT

A core consideration in generating impact is how recommendations are structured and targeted. Recommendations must be clear, evidence-based, and directed to those with the power to act.

In the pilot, recommendations were tailored for:

- Host organisations (e.g., community care departments).
- Sending institutions (e.g., the home university).
- Partner colleges (e.g., vocational training institutions).
- Policymakers (e.g., regional councils, professional regulators).

This stratified approach ensures each actor understands their role in the system-wide improvements recommended by the evaluation. For example, the recommendation to co-develop a structured learning plan was aimed at both the local authority and the academic institution. This dual accountability supports collaboration and shared ownership of future improvements.

MAPPING IMPACT PATHWAYS

The case study provides a useful model for identifying how evaluation findings can influence different layers of policy and practice. Key impact pathways included:

1. **Operational Improvements**: Immediate changes to student induction, placement planning, and mentor engagement emerged as practice-level responses to evaluation insights.
2. **Policy Refinement**: Discussions initiated through the evaluation led to reconsideration of whether vocational qualifications such as the National Vocational Qualification (NVQ) were appropriate for international students. This prompted wider dialogue on qualification equivalency and the suitability of vocational assessment frameworks in transnational contexts.
3. **Institutional Learning**: The home university used the evaluation to reflect on how to best prepare students for international placements, including cultural orientation and communication skills training.
4. **Strategic Partnership Development**: At a higher policy level, the evaluation helped position the pilot as a proof of concept for future international collaborations. Key stakeholders began developing formalised exchange agreements and broader European partnerships.

The ability of an evaluation to influence across these multiple domains depends on the evaluators' capacity to identify who needs to hear what—and when.

BUILDING IMPLEMENTATION INTO THE EVALUATION DESIGN

One common pitfall in programme evaluation is to treat implementation of recommendations as an afterthought. This case study illustrates the value of embedding implementation thinking into the evaluation process from the outset.

A Steering Group of stakeholders—ranging from project leads to academic supervisors and placement managers—was established at the evaluation's inception. This group was not merely advisory; it functioned as a policy translation mechanism. Its role included:

- Reviewing interim findings.
- Validating emerging recommendations.
- Planning for how changes would be actioned after the final report.

By involving those responsible for enacting change in the evaluation process itself, the evaluation team fostered a culture of shared responsibility. This enhanced both the legitimacy and the likelihood of follow-through on recommendations.

USING EVIDENCE TO SUPPORT SYSTEM-LEVEL LEARNING

To move from local practice changes to broader system learning, evaluators must identify generalisable lessons. In the International Placement Pilot Project, this meant distilling insights into themes that resonated beyond the immediate context.

For instance, while the project was geographically specific, its challenges—unclear placement expectations, inconsistent qualification recognition, and limited communication between partners—are common across many international placement initiatives. By framing recommendations in terms of systems learning (e.g., the importance of pre-placement orientation across all transnational programs), the evaluation extended its relevance beyond the immediate pilot project.

System-level learning also requires evidence to be presented in multiple formats. In addition to a full report, the evaluation team developed:

- Executive summaries tailored to different stakeholder audiences.
- Visual diagrams (e.g., process maps) to illustrate partnership mechanisms.
- Thematic analyses highlighting transferable lessons.

This Strategic Communication Approach maximises the accessibility and uptake of findings.

TIMING AND FOLLOW-UP: MAKING RECOMMENDATIONS STICK

Timing is critical when aiming to influence policy and practice. Findings must be delivered when stakeholders are receptive and when budgets, planning cycles, or reform agendas allow space for change.

In the case study, the evaluation report was delivered just as the host organisation was reviewing its recruitment strategy. This meant that evidence from the project could directly inform policy discussions on international workforce development. Similarly, the sending university was in the process of reviewing its curriculum, allowing it to integrate lessons on practice learning into its degree design.

Follow-up is equally important. The evaluation team facilitated post-report debriefings with stakeholders, ensuring recommendations were not only read but discussed and actioned. Ongoing dialogue helped maintain momentum and allowed for iterative adaptation of implementation strategies.

MANAGING COMPLEXITY AND UNINTENDED CONSEQUENCES

Evaluations that aim to influence policy and practice must contend with complexity and unintended outcomes. Not all impacts will be those that were planned or desired. For instance, the requirement for students to complete a vocational qualification (NVQ) was meant to provide structure and recognition. However, it instead led to frustration among students who viewed it as misaligned with their academic trajectory.

This underscores the importance of reflective evaluation practices. Instead of simply noting that students did not complete the NVQ, the evaluation explored why this was the case—highlighting misalignment between institutional expectations and student motivations. This insight has implications for future qualification planning and international partnership negotiations.

Evaluators should embrace such unintended consequences as learning opportunities, not as evaluation weaknesses. Capturing and analysing these dynamics deepens understanding and enhances the credibility of recommendations.

ETHICAL CONSIDERATIONS AND POWER DYNAMICS

When influencing policy and practice, evaluators must navigate ethical tensions and power imbalances. In transnational projects, this includes recognising disparities between sending and receiving countries, as well as, institutional and student-level asymmetries.

In this evaluation, evaluators were acutely aware of possible risks of reproducing unfair dynamics—such as international students being seen as potential low-cost labour. The evaluation deliberately included student voices, gathered through focus groups and questionnaires, to ensure their perspectives informed findings.

This participatory approach not only enhanced ethical rigour but also improved the practical value of the evaluation. By listening to students' critiques—particularly around placement roles, academic support, and cultural adaptation—the evaluation generated recommendations that were grounded in lived experience.

INDICATORS OF POLICY AND PRACTICE IMPACT

How can we tell whether an evaluation has had an impact? Indicators may include:

- Adoption of recommendations into revised programme guidelines.
- Changes to institutional policies (e.g., qualification requirements or induction processes).
- Budget allocations aligned with evaluation priorities.
- Initiation of new partnerships.
- Replication of the pilot model adopted and used more widely.
- Citation of evaluation findings in policy documents or professional standards.

In the pilot evaluation, several such indicators were present. For example, partner organisations began designing more formalised induction processes and considering alternative assessment methods for international placements. Moreover, lessons from the evaluation fed into broader discussions about the role of international students in meeting workforce shortages.

Evaluators should anticipate these potential impacts and plan for ways to monitor them over time, even beyond the formal evaluation period.

LESSONS FOR FUTURE EVALUATORS

Drawing from the experience of the international student placement evaluation, future evaluators can enhance their policy and practice influence by:

1. **Engaging Stakeholders Early**: Involve those who will implement changes from the beginning.
2. **Targeting Recommendations**: Tailor suggestions to specific audiences, using appropriate language and formats.
3. **Embedding Implementation Thinking**: Consider not just what should change, but how and by whom.
4. **Valuing Unintended Learning**: Investigate and learn from unexpected results.
5. **Framing for Generalisability**: Make findings transferable to other settings without losing specificity.
6. **Following-Up**: Plan debriefs and check-ins post-report to support uptake.
7. **Communicating Strategically**: Use multiple channels and formats to reach diverse audiences.

CONCLUSION: FROM INSIGHT TO INFLUENCE

Evaluating impact on policy and practice requires evaluators to bridge evidence and action. It is not enough to measure whether a programme worked; evaluators must also consider how to support meaningful change based on what was learned.

The evaluation of the international social work student placement illustrates that such influence is possible when programme evaluation is designed with purpose, delivered with clarity, and followed through with commitment. By focusing on the connections between learning and doing, evaluators can ensure their work extends beyond the page into improved systems, enhanced practice, and ultimately, better outcomes for all stakeholders involved.

CHAPTER 15

Publications and research

Unlocking the research potential of programme evaluation through a case study of a clinical leadership initiative in a healthcare setting

FROM EVALUATION REPORT TO PUBLICATION: REALISING THE BROADER IMPACT OF EVALUATION RESEARCH

A well-constructed programme evaluation most often concludes with a comprehensive final report serving as both a record of the evaluation process and a key artefact of the knowledge produced. However, the impact of such reports need not end with their delivery to stakeholders. When the evaluation touches on innovative programming, demonstrates novel methods or yields insights with broader relevance, there is considerable potential to disseminate findings more widely through formal publication.

Evaluation reports frequently contain content of interest beyond their immediate context, especially when the programme under review is novel, has achieved notable results or exemplifies an effective use of methodology. For this reason, evaluators and commissioners should consider making reports available in the public domain where they can inform practice and policy elsewhere. Assigning ISBN numbers and uploading reports to institutional repositories or online platforms ensures wider accessibility and permanence, enhancing both visibility and utility.

Beyond report dissemination, the potential for academic or professional publication should be seriously considered. Deriving a peer-reviewed article from an evaluation report can significantly extend the reach of its findings. This is particularly feasible when the evaluation has methodological originality—such as the use of mixed-methods frameworks like the Evaluation Trident—or when the programme evaluated introduces an innovative approach to service delivery. The Trident model,

DOI: 10.4324/9781003312253-15

which incorporates outcomes, processes, and multiple stakeholder perspectives provides fertile ground for reflection on evaluation design itself, which may appeal to methodological journals.

Moreover, many evaluation studies feature components that, while not central to the overall report, are nonetheless suitable for thematic publication. For instance, evaluators may publish a standalone paper focusing on a conceptual framework developed during the evaluation, such as a model of supervision or engagement, a new approach to stakeholder feedback, or adaptations to mixed-method data integration. By selecting and elaborating on such components, evaluators can create focused publications that contribute to ongoing disciplinary debates or applied practitioner knowledge.

The path to publication requires intentional planning. Each prospective journal—whether aimed at academic audiences or practitioner readership—has its own submission guidelines, stylistic preferences, and conceptual orientations. Evaluators are advised to carefully study the scope, tone, and structure of published articles in targeted journals before drafting their submission. Doing so not only ensures compliance with formal requirements but also increases the likelihood that the submission will resonate with the journal's editorial priorities.

In addition to supporting knowledge dissemination and sector-wide learning, publishing the results of a programme evaluation can contribute meaningfully to professional development. Engaging in the publication process enhances evaluators' and programme staff's research and writing skills, supports academic promotion or career advancement, and strengthens institutional credibility. For evaluation, teams based within universities or other research organisations such as publications may also feed into broader research programs, curriculum development, or future funding proposals.

The connection between programme evaluation and the social and behavioural sciences further strengthens its publication potential. Evaluation draws on a wide range of disciplinary tools—from ethnography and interviews to statistical modelling and realist synthesis—making it an adaptable platform for interdisciplinary publication. When linked to answering applied evaluation questions, these methods are often reframed in dynamic and accessible ways that can appeal to a broad academic audience. Evaluation research can, therefore, become a bridge between methodological innovation and applied policy work, making it particularly valuable to journals that seek to straddle theory and practice.

From an educational standpoint, involving staff and stakeholders in the development of a publishable product can be highly beneficial. The process of converting a report into an article demands reflection, synthesis, and conceptual framing, which can deepen participants' understanding of both the subject matter and the practice of evaluation itself. For educators, integrating such real-world evaluation outputs into research methods courses not only brings vitality to teaching but also builds the evaluation capacity of future practitioners.

Case Study: An Evaluation of a Clinical Leadership Initiative in a healthcare setting

Programme evaluations often culminate in final reports that summarise findings, propose recommendations, and serve the commissioning organisation's internal needs. However, the scope of impact for a well-executed evaluation can extend far beyond internal reporting. When conceived and documented with academic rigour, evaluations can contribute to wider discourses in social and behavioural research and lay the groundwork for future publications. This chapter explores how to develop and disseminate evaluation findings using the evaluation of a clinical leadership initiative in a healthcare setting as a case study.

THE PUBLICATION OF FINAL REPORTS AND RESEARCH-READY EVALUATIONS

One of the most immediate outputs of a programme evaluation is the final report. While often written with practitioners and commissioners in mind, the report can also serve as a stepping stone for further dissemination through research publications, conference presentations, and professional learning materials. To serve both practical and academic audiences, evaluators should write with clarity, evidence, and a consistent methodological framework from the outset.

In this case study, the use of the Trident Evaluation Model enabled the evaluators to organise findings in a manner suitable for both operational learning and academic analysis. The final report structure, with clearly delineated sections on outcomes, processes, and multiple stakeholder perspectives, offered a natural basis for thematically driven publications.

A key to future publication lies in preserving and archiving qualitative data systematically. Transcribed interviews, coding frameworks, thematic analyses, and participant narratives can be anonymised and revisited for secondary analysis. In this case, interviews were conducted with a variety of participants providing rich material that revealed tensions between the aspirations of the model and its practical implementation. These datasets are valuable for further theorising leadership, team-based practice, or implementation of science.

EVALUATION AS SOCIAL AND BEHAVIOURAL RESEARCH

When evaluations are approached through the lens of social and behavioural research they can offer insights far beyond the programme in question. They provide real-world sites for examining organisational change, professional identity, leadership, motivation, communication, and policy translation.

This case study, for instance, did not merely assess whether the system of clinical leaders in healthcare settings was functioning. It revealed layers of professional dynamics: how roles are adopted or resisted, how knowledge is disseminated (or not), and how institutional memory fades when initiatives lose organisational support.

Several findings exemplify key concepts in organisational behaviour and health service research. These include:

- **Role Ambiguity and Identity**: Many expressed uncertainty about the boundaries and responsibilities of the clinical leadership role. This ambiguity is a rich area for further research into professional identity formation and the implementation of change initiatives.
- **Motivational Misalignment**: Assigning staff to leadership areas without consultation undermined intrinsic motivation—a topic well explored in self-determination theory but underexamined in healthcare evaluation contexts.
- **Barriers to Knowledge Translation**: Despite the initial infrastructure—training, literature access, meetings—many leaders lacked time and ongoing support, which highlights systemic issues around knowledge mobilisation in practice settings.

These are all areas ripe for academic inquiry using established behavioural science frameworks. The qualitative data already collected for the case study could be recoded or reanalysed to answer more specific theoretical questions, perhaps, in collaboration with academic researchers.

OPPORTUNITIES FOR ACADEMIC AND PROFESSIONAL PUBLICATIONS

Programme evaluation reports are often viewed as grey literature—documents that, while informative, lack the academic polish required for peer-reviewed journals. Yet many contain findings of significant interest to disciplinary and interdisciplinary fields. By reframing the purpose and audience, evaluators can transform findings into publishable research outputs.

Journals and outlets

Depending on the focus of the evaluation, possible publication venues include:

- *Health and Social Care in the Community.*
- *Evaluation.*
- *Journal of Advanced Nursing.*
- *Public Administration Review.*
- *Educational Evaluation and Policy Analysis.*
- *Leadership in Health Services.*

Each journal has distinct expectations. For example, a submission to *Evaluation* might require a methodological reflection on the use of the Trident model, while *Leadership in Health Services* might welcome a focused discussion on the implementation challenges of distributed leadership models.

In this case study, a particularly strong candidate for publication is a thematic paper on professional role construction and leadership in clinical teams. By focusing on qualitative data from multiple stakeholder groups, the paper could contribute to the literature on team functioning, innovation implementation, and nursing leadership.

Thematic focus areas for publication

Some potential themes drawn from the case study include:

- **Implementation Failure and Organisational Memory**: How well-intentioned initiatives decline over time.
- **The Hidden Curriculum in Clinical Teams**: Unwritten rules and implicit knowledge transfer in specialty teams.
- **Communication Strategies and Discontinuities**: Evaluating tools such as ward communication folders and notice boards.
- **Barriers to Research Engagement among Practitioners**: Examining why a limited number were involved in original research during the implementation phase.
- **Reintroducing Named Roles in Fragmented Systems**: A comparison of old and new models of healthcare continuity.

Each of these could be explored through additional literature review and possibly further data collection, if resources allow.

ETHICAL CONSIDERATIONS FOR SECONDARY USE OF DATA

When intending to publish beyond the initial evaluation ethical concerns need to be revisited. Evaluations typically follow audit or service improvement protocols that may not meet the standard for academic research ethics approval. To publish in peer-reviewed journals, especially where participants are quoted or analysed in depth, one of two pathways is usually followed:

- **Seek Retrospective Ethical Approval**: Some institutions allow for ethics review of pre-collected data, especially if it was anonymised and participants gave informed consent for future use.
- **Design Future Evaluations with Dual Purpose**: Evaluators intending to publish should design their data collection and consent processes with this dual purpose in mind. This includes clarifying with participants that their anonymised data may be used for research and publication.

EMBEDDING EVALUATIONS IN RESEARCH PROGRAMS

One way to bridge the gap between evaluation and research is to embed evaluations within broader research programs or academic-practice partnerships. This allows for:

- Longitudinal follow-up.
- Comparative studies across sites or agencies.
- Development of theory-informed intervention models.
- Contributions to mixed-method research methodologies.

This case study provides a foundation for follow-up studies particularly if future iterations of the leadership model are implemented. Evaluators could return to the same unit to assess changes in perceptions, role clarity, and outcomes, creating a valuable longitudinal data set.

Moreover, in this instance, thematic networks developed through qualitative coding could serve as the basis for more complex comparative work across other units, programs, or institutions. These networks offer conceptual frames for testing or further refining theoretical propositions in behavioural and social science.

CREATING A DISSEMINATION STRATEGY

To maximise the reach and impact of a programme evaluation, the following dissemination steps are advisable:

1. **Internal Debriefings and Workshops**: Use evaluation results to lead reflective practice sessions within host organisations.
2. **Summary Reports for Professional Bodies**: Translate findings into practical recommendations tailored to professional audiences.
3. **Conference Papers and Posters**: National or international conferences in health services, education, social work, or public policy are ideal platforms to present early findings and build academic interest.
4. **Journal Submissions**: Prepare at least one paper based on key themes.
5. **Digital Repositories**: Host anonymised reports and summaries in institutional or subject-specific open-access repositories to broaden reach.

PRACTICAL TIPS FOR TURNING EVALUATION INTO RESEARCH

To support evaluators seeking to expand their work into publishable research, the following steps are recommended:

- **Use a Recognised Evaluation Framework**: Models like the Trident are especially helpful for translating practice-based evaluation into research-ready formats.
- **Document Methodology Transparently**: Describe your data collection and analysis processes clearly and thoroughly in your evaluation report.
- **Archive Raw Data Securely**: Maintain anonymised transcripts and coded data in line with institutional and legal requirements.
- **Think Thematically**: From the outset, consider potential theoretical contributions or disciplinary debates your evaluation may inform.
- **Collaborate with Academic Partners**: This brings methodological rigour and publication experience.
- **Be Realistic About Time**: Translating evaluation into publication requires time and commitment beyond the project timeline.
- **Secure Consent for Publication**: Even if anonymised participants should be informed that data might be used for research dissemination.

CONCLUSION: EVALUATION AS A RESEARCH-GENERATING ACTIVITY

Thoughtfully conducted programme evaluations offer more than assessments on effectiveness—they are opportunities for organisational learning, stakeholder reflection, and long-term strategic development. One of the most important lessons emerging from the case study is that the impact of evaluation depends not just on findings but on how those findings are used and communicated.

A key practical insight is the importance of integrating publication planning into the evaluation process from the outset. Rather than waiting until the final report is written, programme evaluators and commissioners should identify components with broader relevance early on—such as innovative methodologies, models of engagement, or unexpected outcomes—and flag them for possible dissemination. Doing this allows time for ethical considerations, additional data analysis, and alignment with potential publication venues.

Another lesson is the value of collaboration throughout the evaluation process. Involving stakeholders in shaping the evaluation questions, interpreting findings, and reviewing draft outputs fosters ownership and increases the likelihood that results will be acted upon. These collaborations can also lay the groundwork for co-authored publications contributing to both the credibility and richness of dissemination efforts.

Practically speaking, programme evaluators must become strategic communicators. This means tailoring outputs to different audiences—producing concise summaries for practitioners, technical papers for academic readers, and accessible visuals for community stakeholders. Investing in this communication work multiplies the usefulness of the programme evaluation and ensures it lives beyond the summative report stage.

The case study also highlighted the need for evaluators to maintain reflective practice. Keeping field notes, evaluation diaries, or internal memos during the project can help capture insights that may not appear in the final report but are valuable for publication, teaching, or future evaluations. These reflective practices encourage evaluators to see their work not just as a product but as a contribution to an evolving field.

Finally, the case study underscores that programme evaluations gain influence when evaluators are proactive in connecting with relevant networks—whether professional associations, academic groups, or policy forums. Sharing learning in these spaces helps to translate local findings into wider application and strengthens the legitimacy of evaluation as a driver of change.

In summation, programme evaluation matters most when it is shared purposefully. The path from programme evaluation to broader influence is not automatic; it requires deliberate planning, reflective engagement, and strategic dissemination. These are not peripheral tasks—they are central to making programme evaluation count.

CHAPTER 16

Conclusion

Programme evaluation as a tool for continuous quality improvement

INTRODUCTION: EMBEDDING EVALUATION INTO CONTINUOUS QUALITY IMPROVEMENT

Programme evaluation is not merely a retrospective judgement on success or failure—it is a vital instrument for ongoing learning, maintaining success, and Continuous Quality Improvement (CQI). By systematically collecting, analysing, and acting on data, evaluations help refine practices, guide resource allocation and generate innovation across services. This chapter outlines how evaluations can be structurally and purposefully embedded into CQI processes, drawing on the Evaluation Trident methodology, which focuses on outcomes, processes, and stakeholder perspectives. It illustrates how this approach enhances organisational learning, service delivery, participant satisfaction, and professional development.

FROM EVALUATION TO IMPROVEMENT: THE CQI MINDSET

Continuous Quality Improvement (CQI) is a structured, ongoing effort to improve service performance, outcomes, and organisational efficiency. It relies on iterative feedback loops in which evaluations serve both diagnostic and developmental roles. A well-structured programme evaluation supports CQI by:

- Assessing whether objectives have been achieved (outcomes).
- Uncovering how implementation aligns with best practice (process).
- Engaging diverse voices to refine future directions (stakeholder perspectives).

Evaluations that are explicitly designed to feed into CQI processes can stimulate measurable and sustainable improvements across multiple domains of service and programme delivery.

DOI: 10.4324/9781003312253-16

REVISITING KEY PRINCIPLES OF PROGRAMME EVALUATION IN CQI

The following foundational principles enable programme evaluation to effectively support CQI:

1. **Purpose-Driven Design**
   Evaluations must begin with clarity of purpose: what are we seeking to improve?
2. **Integration with Organisational Strategy**
   Evaluations should align with broader institutional goals and national standards.
3. **Use of Multi-Source Evidence**
   Combining anecdotal, documentary, and observational data ensures a comprehensive view of success and areas for enhancement.
4. **Reflexivity and Learning Orientation**
   A Learning-Focused Approach acknowledges complexity and adapts methods and focus areas over time.

APPLYING THE TRIDENT EVALUATION FOR CONTINUOUS QUALITY IMPROVEMENT

The Trident Evaluation Model encompasses three key areas:

A. Outcomes: Are Stated Objectives Being Met?

Evaluation involves tracking objectives related to development, training, service improvement, and organisational growth. Combining multiple data sources helps assess whether objectives are met, in progress, or incomplete. Unmet objectives offer valuable insight for adaptive planning.

Tip: Use a structured tracking sheet for annual objectives with status columns for completion, barriers, and follow-up action. Regular review sessions should be embedded in organisational routines.

B. Process: How Was the Programme Delivered?

Mapping internal processes illuminates how ideas progress from concept to implementation. A typical project cycle may involve:

1. Identifying a problem or service need.
2. Reviewing relevant evidence.
3. Auditing current practice.
4. Implementing change.
5. Evaluating outcomes.
6. Disseminating findings.

Not every project follows the full cycle but a transparent model enables visualisation of pathways to improvement.

Tip: Articulate and visualise a "theory of change" or a realistic model at the outset. Revisit it at each stage to ensure alignment between intentions and delivery.

C. Stakeholder Perspectives: What Did People Think?

Through structured interviews and thematic analysis, evaluations capture insights from practitioners, participants, educators, and managers. Themes often include:

- Value of interprofessional collaboration.
- Challenges in maintaining engagement.
- Impact on individual development and morale.
- Communication gaps across organisational boundaries.

These narratives offer a deeper understanding of the dynamics that influence implementation and outcomes.

Tip: Stakeholder feedback should not be tokenistic. Build structured spaces—forums, listening sessions, feedback loops—into project timelines. Use qualitative data analysis tools to explore and elevate emergent themes.

TRANSLATING EVALUATION INTO ACTION: CQI IN PRACTICE

A key feature of successful evaluations is a commitment to *acting on findings*. Insights should directly inform:

- Development and revision of training and education initiatives.
- Strategic decisions on resource allocation.
- Prioritisation of service improvement areas.
- Enhanced integration of evidence into routine protocols.

Each evaluation cycle should contribute to an evolving agenda, reinforcing a culture of reflection, learning, and responsive action.

Tip: Publish a concise annual CQI report highlighting "changes made as a result of evaluation." This reinforces the message that evaluation is not an endpoint but a catalyst. Be sure to promote changes and success which maintains interest and engagement.

CHALLENGES AND LESSONS LEARNED

Common challenges encountered in embedding evaluation into CQI include:

- **Sustaining Momentum**: Staff turnover and limited administrative support can undermine continuity.
- **Balancing Roles**: Tensions may arise between operational, educational, and research commitments.
- **Evaluation Fatigue**: Staff and participants may perceive evaluations as burdensome especially when feedback is not visibly acted upon.

Recommendations should include streamlining administrative processes, clarifying project roles, and embedding micro-evaluation into daily practice.

THE ROLE OF EVALUATION IN ORGANISATIONAL LEARNING

Beyond project assessment, evaluations support **organisational learning**. They help reveal patterns, enable strategic pivoting, and foster a culture of inquiry.

For example, evaluations showing low participation in certain initiatives may prompt redesigns, while gaps in research capacity may lead to mentorship schemes or collaboration.

Tip: Don't discard "negative" results. Use them as springboards for inquiry: why didn't it work? What conditions would enable success next time?

RECOMMENDATIONS FOR EMBEDDING CQI EVALUATION

The following recommendations are offered for those seeking to embed evaluation in CQI:

1. **Make Evaluation Routine**: Integrate it into the regular service/programme cycle.
2. **Align with Strategic Goals**: Focus on evaluation questions that reflect priority areas.
3. **Foster Multi-Level Engagement**: Engage stakeholders from design to dissemination.
4. **Use Mixed Methods Thoughtfully**: Combine quantitative data with qualitative data and insights.
5. **Invest in Capacity Building**: Provide staff with training in evaluation and data analysis.

CONCLUSION: EVALUATION AS AN ENGINE OF IMPROVEMENT

Programme evaluations, when intentionally integrated into CQI systems, become engines for transformation. They support innovation, strengthen accountability, and nurture a culture of shared responsibility for improvement

In conclusion, programme evaluation, when properly embedded in CQI efforts, becomes much more than an accountability tool. It evolves into a continuous source of feedback, learning, and improvement. Organisations that embrace evaluation as part of their culture are better equipped to adapt to change, meet stakeholder needs, and deliver high-quality, effective programs and services. Rather than an end-of-cycle reflection, evaluation becomes a continuous dialogue between data, practice, and vision.

As this guide has outlined, the principles and practices of programme evaluation are not only methodologically sound and practically achievable—they are powerful tools for driving meaningful change. When thoughtfully applied, evaluation can strengthen services, inform policy, and empower communities, ultimately contributing to a more just, inclusive, and healthier society.

Index

Note: Page numbers in *italics* refer to figures.

For Product Safety Concerns and Information please contact our
EU representative GPSR@taylorandfrancis.com Taylor & Francis
Verlag GmbH, Kaufingerstraße 24, 80331 München, Germany